nobility (n.)

the state of being in one's

character, mind, birthright, rank.

Associated with

dignity, goodness and

courage.

The *Joy* of NURSING

Reclaiming Our Nobility

Steamboat Springs Publishing

Juliana Adams
BSN, MSN, MA

Steamboat Springs Publishing

Books may be purchased in bulk by contacting the publisher or author:
Email: SteamboatSpringsPublishing@gmail.com
Webpage: SteamboatSpringsPublishing.com

Cover Painting: Kimberly Conrad, www.KimberlyConradFineArt.com
Cover and Interior Design: Rebecca Finkel, F + P Graphic Design
Editing: Melanie Stafford
Publisher: Steamboat Springs Publishing
Creative Consultant: Judith Briles, The Book Shepherd

Library of Congress Catalog Number 2016930482
978-0-9972003-0-0 (soft cover)
978-0-9972003-2-4 (hard cover)
978-0-9972003-1-7 (ebook)

1. Nursing   2. Management   3. Inspiration   4. Health

First Edition
Printed in USA

We All Enter This World

We all enter this world with the entrusted life work

To fulfill our own unique destiny.

Our life's purpose may not be known to us,

But like water flowing around rocks in a stream,

We are all challenged to see beyond the known visible boundaries,

In search of deeper meanings within ourselves.

Could we not have a more sacred journey?

To seek to understand and find meaning,

To what is often simply called,

"The mystery of life?"

—Juliana Adams, 2011

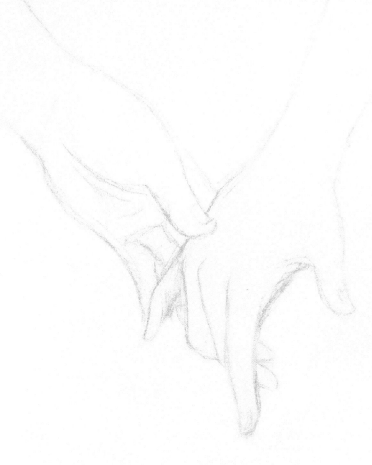

To my nursing friends and colleagues

that have chosen the

laying on of hands,

in service to another ...

Believing

that the profession of nursing is noble,

because of the patients

who trust us to care for them.

Contents

Foreword

*J*uliana Adams' *The Joy of Nursing* touched my heart and soul, stirring up embedded memories of what nursing is, and should be. If it wasn't for a nurse, one Sylvia Eaton RN, my three children would have been orphaned at the ages of 10, 12 and 13 in April of 1976.

Being told by my regular physician that it was "just monthly female issues" that would go away and to "just go back to work;" and then being told by another doctor that I really didn't need to see anyone else and was "wasting my time asking for another appointment," didn't feel right. I wasn't a medical doctor; I believed them. The appointment I had made with "yet another doctor" was cancelled by me when my doctor told me my pain could be because of kidney stones and he would schedule tests the following week. My gnawing lower belly pain persisted.

My pain resonated with RN Sylvia Eaton. She called me back an hour after I had cancelled my slated appointment. She recited what I had said my complaints were, pushing me to reschedule—as in get to her doctor's office that day. I heard her; my head heard her and my body told me, "Leave work now and meet this new doctor."

Two hours later, I sat across from him, telling him my story. He was alarmed and alert as he told me that I needed emergency surgery. She remained by my side till I was transferred to the hospital.

Days turned into weeks. The toxicity in my body from the Dalkon Shield IUD created an epic battlefield for a team of surgeons who had to deal with a ruptured colon and bladder. I arrested while in surgery and did not leave the hospital until a month later. I had more tubes and gadgets attached to my body than I could imagine, and I was angry at not being listened to until Sylvia looked at me and listened to me. Because of her, I had gone in to be seen instead of giving up.

My recovery took many months. The unhooking and removal of all the gizmos and gadgets was welcomed by my body.

- If it hadn't been for Sylvia Eaton's nursing experience, her intuitiveness, her unexpected follow-up—let's say outright hounding—and yes, her caring ... I wouldn't be alive today.

- If it hadn't been for her nobility—the character, dignity, goodness and courage to speak up and out, to take charge with someone that she had only connected with via the telephone, and again when I came in to be seen ... I wouldn't be alive today.

Nurses have saved patients lives for many years in our hospitals, clinics, offices, in home care, over the phone and increasingly now by advancing and advocating for innovative and new ways to promote health and caring. They are our guardian angels—sometimes very visibly; sometimes "just there" with their eyes and ears.

Little did I know that I would dedicate 20 years of my life as an expert in toxic behaviors in the health care industry years later. My experience as a patient seeded multiple national studies and the publishing of several books dealing with conflict in the workplace.

Within *The Joy of Nursing, Reclaiming Our Nobility* you will meet one of those guardian angels, Juliana Adams. Her stories, her insights, and her dedication to nursing spanning 50 years are exactly what exhausted, overwhelmed, disillusioned, naïve and those entering nursing need today. Some of her stories, the situations she reveals and insights that only decades can deliver, will break your heart; some will alarm you; and some will have you standing and cheering. Juliana is an RN, a "real nurse," whose candid revealing will make you feel safer and more cared for.

She relates exciting "Camelot" experiences and those that were not. What she learned at the toughest of places provided her with the desire to seek a deeper understanding of what being a nurse was all about. Discovering where the nobility of nursing came from was inspiring to me, a non nurse. To those nurses presently working, it will be revitalizing.

Nursing, and its nobility, is at the core of a healthy and vibrant health care system. *The Joy of Nursing* will rekindle the nursing spirit that is the essence of healing care. We all should thank those who enter its doors and remind those they work for how vital they are.

—JUDITH BRILES, DBA, MBA
Stabotage: How to Deal with the Pit Bulls,
Skunks, Snakes, Scorpions and Slugs
in the Health Care Workplace

Preface

"I'm your nurse today,
and I will be here for you to make things better."

I didn't start out saying this to patients in my early years. All new nurses, from before my time in the 1960s, to the present, travel along a similar path of feeling overwhelmed until their education, skills and nursing acumen does become who they are.

My fifty-year nursing career began with dreams based on very little reality, but I did become a "real nurse." By my tenth year or so, my "expert years" began. These years revealed to me that there was more to the nurse/patient relationship than the care that I gave to patients. I realized that there were more similarities to the reasons *why* and *who* decided to become a nurse throughout the last five decades, than there were differences.

What has and what has not changed since Florence Nightingale's time for the women and men that feel called to be nurses?

No one wants to be a patient, but few of us live life without having to, at some time, find ourselves needing the "kindness of an intimate stranger:" a nurse. Finding my own "roadmap of being," desiring to discover my own sacred story of transformations through the years, took place to some degree, in every position I have held as a nurse.

I never felt like I had done it all, even as the years went by. ICUs, ERs, Community Health, Ambulatory Care, starting a home care business for seniors, interwoven with positions in leadership, academia and research—in private and for-profit organizations that were small, big, magnet, unionized and struggling environments both in Europe and America—were all part of my curriculum vitae. I experienced "Camelot Nursing." I experienced environments, positions and people that educated, inspired and broadened my understanding of what nurses could do. I was never "just a nurse." Not all my positions were easy but going to work was never a drudge; I believed that I made a difference. For the first 25 years I was not concerned with perceptions of nursing or proving my value. As more layers of staff were added, and held the title of "nurse," what to expect from a nurse was confusing.

As I look back, it makes me smile as I think of events that exceeded anything that I could have imagined. The colorful stories are pieces of my shimmery mosaic life that has never been dull. Leah Curtain, a Grand Dame within nursing for the last sixty years, invites nurses to make the conscious choice of being "present" with patients, by bringing an attitude of "healing mental energy." *Any given moment—no matter how casual, how ordinary—is poised, full of gaping life.—* Anne Michaels

To do something for fifty years—what did I learn along the way?

Exposure to toughness but holding on to being gentle and compassionate is a familiar dilemma for most nurses at some point in their careers. Nurses are "comfortable being uncomfortable" my nurse friend Marion told me two decades ago. This discomfort, this frustration occurs more often in regards to the environment where nursing is practiced than in regards to the care nurses deliver with their peers. The profession of nursing is strong enough for us all to nudge, poke and prod it.

Inviting dialogues of discontent is valuable, necessary and has to be respected and available to all of us to participate in. This ensures that academia, leadership and the hands-on nurses' perspective create solutions that work for all of us.

Nobility is a word that you don't hear that often today in regards to many professions. Corny, excessive, idealistic or hyperbole might come to mind. Nursing has ranked as the "most trusted profession" in diverse surveys of the public's perception on trust and respect, but how does this fit with what else you've heard or personally experienced as a nurse, non-nurse or patient?

I would expect a Boomer and a Millennial nurse to have differences of opinions, and yet bonding between the four generations of nurses currently practicing today is less of an issue than our mutual concerns with those that employ us.

Historically, the purpose of a Preface is to "explain, apologize or to defend" the ideas that were to follow in the book. I could not have written *The Joy of Nursing, Reclaiming Our Nobility* if I had not experienced the complex, non-ideal work environment of the last decade. Reclaiming the carative art and joy of nursing did occur and provided me with closure, resulting in the confidence that my nursing experience was not singular to me alone. Sharing "uncomfortable truths instead of obscuring them allows that beneath shiny surfaces, there lies a different type of beauty."

Much of what nurses do remains unclear to those outside of the profession. The depth, diversity and richness I present is through the eyes of a young "Blue Angel" volunteer to the present, spanning fifty years of practice. This book was written from the perspective of narrative-cultural knowledge. It is intended for those considering becoming a nurse and nurses presently practicing who may have become disillusioned along the way. Rediscovering the joy of being a nurse occurred paradoxically at a time in my career that I considered the job I was in, to be the least satisfying.

Sharing uncomfortable truths
instead of obscuring them allows that
Beneath shiny surfaces,
there lies a different type of beauty.

—KRISTA BREMER, associate publisher, *The Sun* magazine

The Joy of Nursing, Reclaiming Our Nobility
is a candid personal story of discovery,
rediscovery, inspiration and joy.

PART I

THE JOY

"Figuring out joy will be a gift for life."

CHAPTER 1

My Magical Beliefs Set the Stage for a Lifetime

People in trouble sought out nurses to talk to because nurses appeared kind, wise, and something else: happy.

Think of the world you carry only within yourself.

had only been a patient once in my life, but it made a lasting impression. I was four years old, living with my family in Germany, where my father, a U.S. Army officer, was stationed. I'd burned my foot when I jumped out of bed early and was running in the hallway of our large drafty house, and a pot of scalding water was on the floor sitting on top of a floor heat register. I had to be flown back to the United States on a military transport plane for treatment.

All of the other patients traveling to Walter Reed Army Medical Center's burn unit were soldiers. I was a little girl with big eyes and too-long bangs. The staff put me in a metal crib with sides too high for me to climb out. I remember how the soldiers drew pictures for me, how they handed me candy bars when the nurses weren't looking, and how my foot had this big fluffy dressing on it.

My parents could not accompany me on the emergency evacuation flight. My mother and twin sister would meet up with me two weeks later, after they took a boat from Germany. Being held by an army nurse in a big blanket and cuddled made me feel not so alone; what could have been a terrifying experience was not.

Later on, I would remember these nurses and my good feelings about them. I had other good feelings when I thought about nurses out in the world. I wanted to be a nurse from the time I was eight years old. I liked what they *did*. They got to be there when the babies were born and when people died. They helped people who were hurting. People in trouble sought out nurses to talk to, because nurses appeared kind, wise, and something else: happy. My young mind concluded that nurses were happy because they were doing something important.

Nurses came in all shapes and sizes. Some were young and pretty, and some looked a little grouchy and like they didn't really care if they were pretty or not, but they all looked like they were proud of themselves. My mother was a stay-at-home mom, and I thought I would never want to stay home every day, even if I loved my children a lot. Our neighbor was our school nurse, and everyone liked and respected her. She told me that I "would make a very dedicated nurse someday." Her comments made me beam.

Nurses made a difference in the world and the patients they treated. I wanted to be one.

I didn't have any relatives who were nurses. I read all the books about nurses I could get my hands on, including the Cherry Ames series, and I learned about Clara Barton. But after I got older, around the sixth grade, I stopped saying I wanted to be like those characters. I wanted to show I was serious about becoming a nurse. The fact that only one of these *girls* was real and one fictional did matter to me. By the mid-1960s, when I was looking seriously at where to attend college, mostly never-married women, divorced women, or widowed women worked. I wasn't sure if they worked out of economic necessity or if they *wanted* to work.

We had a healthy family. I realized that I had no experience with sickness, suffering or death with the exception of my burned foot experience. Disease, sadness, fear, or how sickness affected one's family was not even imaginable to me because the occasional nurse I saw on TV usually looked ready to do something, I just wasn't sure what.

In high school in the Bay Area of California, I was aware of the women's movement, and even though I had heard the idea that young women could be "more than teachers and nurses," I knew nursing was not a "default" career for me. It would take a decade before I was aware that being a nurse might not be quite as romantic as the nurses in the movies *A Farewell to Arms* or *In Harm's Way*, but I never saw or read anything to make me question that the nursing image I had was too idealistic. It wouldn't have mattered by then!

At 14, no more waiting! I became a Blue Angel in the local veterans' hospital and began to earnestly observe and listen to the nurses I eagerly assisted.

If one is lucky, one solitary fantasy can totally transform one million realities.

— MAYA ANGELOU

CHAPTER 2

It All Started with a Lie to a Nun

I believed that I would know when I had
this special relationship with patients,
however brief at first, but that I would be
this wise, kind woman like Flo [Nightingale].

*Service is the rent we pay for
the privilege of living on this earth.*

Bustling across the street from my dorm at
Providence College of Nursing in Oakland,
California, I wrapped my long, navy-blue nurse's
cape around me against the cold. The smell of oatmeal and frying
bacon stopped me for a minute as I stood still between two
brick buildings, my dorm and Providence Hospital. I was 19,
slim, bright-eyed, and utterly and delightfully alive. Attending
a three-year diploma school after attending college was, even
in 1968, an old-fashioned way to become a nurse, but it felt
perfect to me—even after my first uncomfortable interview with
the Catholic sisters two days before the application deadline.

I had no time to think about my answers to the questions Sister Elizabeth Ann might ask at my formal interview, but I knew that I had been working on why I wanted to be a nurse for a lifetime.

"So, Juliana, what religion are you?" Sister Elizabeth Ann asked me as soon as I sat down in her office.

What religion am I? It never occurred to me that she would ask me God questions. Looking up, I answered, "Protestant."

"Yes, dear, that is what you wrote in your application. What type of Protestant are you?"

What type of Protestant? Wasn't that good enough? Looking down, I answered, "Lutheran."

After the interview I went out to join my parents, who were sitting in the car waiting for me. ("We don't want you to drive to Oakland; it's too dangerous.") I asked my dad what religion we were, and he said, "Protestant." I then asked him what type of Protestant, and he replied, "Methodist."

I looked at him, looking at me in the rearview mirror, and said, "Not any more. We're now officially Lutheran."

Hurry up, Juliana, I thought to myself. *Get going or you won't have time to check on your two assigned patients for the day before the nuns come around and ask you a question that you only vaguely know the answer to.* I was starving, and breakfast was the best meal of the day in the hospital's basement cafeteria, so get going I did.

Within just a few months of schooling here at this 100-year-old nursing school, it reinforced what I had always known, that I wanted only to be a nurse. How else could I explain that I even found wearing the white stockings and plain, white, shapeless novice uniform less distasteful than I said it was to my non-nurse friends. In fact, I even loved the clunky white shoes that required so much work each night to polish and wash out the laces, hoping the polish wouldn't rub off the shoes onto my hands, requiring yet another coat of the sticky, white goo.

Having only two hospital days the first semester meant only two 5:00 a.m. wakeups, which even for me, an early riser, still felt cold and dark in December. I dressed quickly in clothes laid out the night before. Entering the hospital before the night nurses left and the day nurses came on felt special to me. I was becoming a part of this group of women: *real nurses*, as my friends and I called the registered nurses (RNs).

This particular morning, I hoped to dodge them all, sheepishly praying that a tired, end-of-the-shift nurse bustling around finishing up her intake and output of fluid totals on her patients (I and O's) wouldn't ask me to dump a bedpan because I needed to get in and get out quickly. If I was waylaid, I knew I would grumble later, but it would go unnoticed because everyone grumbled a lot. I grumbled, but I was happy in this cloistered life so different from my home growing up in Palo Alto, California.

Unlike other young women in the mid-1960s, I did have other career choices. It actually took courage for me to say that I wanted to be a nurse, when in my family, being a doctor would not have been considered unusual. How lucky I was that I had parents who never said "Is that all you want to be, a nurse?" My parents were, however, concerned about my choice to go to Oakland, California, to "Pill Hill" where indigent care was delivered by two out of the three hospitals on this knoll in downtown Oakland.

Get going, Juliana!

During the first semester of school, Sister Elizabeth Ann introduced Florence Nightingale to all 40 of us. "A shining example of the nobility of nursing," was how this smooth-faced nun, who never really smiled or frowned, described "Flo," as my more irreverent classmates would call this famous nurse.

Up until then, my image of her was probably the same as that of any young, wannabe nurse in the United States: some selfless girl who never got married and instead went around and bandaged up soldiers on battlefields and got famous for it. She was noble. She didn't care about catching diseases; she just did for others.

All of the above, I learned, was more or less true, but there was a whole lot more to Flo's story.

She was "a ministering angel," I remember writing down, even if I wasn't quite sure what this meant. She was introduced to us all as the founder of modern nursing. She elevated the practice of nursing to a level of professionalism never considered before her time. I read and heard this in a course most likely called the History of Nursing. From all I learned about her then and since, I think it's safe to say *she* never would have considered herself noble. Years of caring for patients resulted in her defining how all aspects of caring for a patient could be improved upon, until her death at age 90.

However, I wouldn't *know* this myself back in 1968, not for years to come.

I never heard anyone speak to the nobility of nursing again for the next 35 years. I did carry within me this beginning vision of nurses as heroines. This vision came to me when I saw a nursing colleague interact with a patient or family whenever she seemed confident, tender, or somehow communicated the message that *everything will be all right.* I tucked into memory the mental image of how I could be *someday.* I believed that I would know when I had this special relationship with patients, however brief at first, but that I would be this wise, kind woman like Flo.

This was a romantic fantasy, but I held onto this personalized vision just as I believed other Catholic nursing students were guided by saints. Images of Nightingale never quite left my heart.

In the years to come, I discovered a lot about what it meant to be a nurse. I began to understand on a more revelatory level what the word "nobility" meant in the context of nursing.

Who was Florence Nightingale?

She was born to wealthy British parents in Florence, Italy, on May 12, 1820, her namesake. When she was one year old, her family moved back to England, and Nightingale was brought up in the family's various gracious homes. An attractive young girl, Nightingale was schooled in literature and mathematics by her father, who believed in the education of women. However, he did not approve, nor did the rest of her family, of Florence choosing not to marry and deciding instead to become a nurse. She then began her education of being a nurse the way all nurses did at the time, by being present on the wards in hospitals, learning by watching and doing.

Florence believed God had "called her to be a nurse." She considered nursing a "calling," a calling, that for her, was in a religious sense. One became a nurse because nurses needed to have "feelings for one's work." She stated that "enthusiasm" (based on the Greek *entheos*, "having the god within") should guide one's decision to be a caregiver.

Despite her mother's anger and society's disapproval, she chose to forego the pursuit of marriageable men. One in particular—a persistent, British politician who courted her for nine years—was ultimately jilted when she left for Crimea in 1853, after England sent soldiers there to fight. She was able to fulfill her desire to go there because of her father's financial support. She went to care for soldiers on the battlefield. The conditions she later recounted, caused her to begin a personal crusade of improving the horrific care soldiers received. It was at this time she became known as the "lady with the lamp," because she remained with her patients throughout the night.

Nightingale came into the public awareness during the Crimean War. She and 28 nurses she trained provided care to soldiers. She confronted military generals regarding the unspeakable conditions soldiers endured. Deaths from mass infections, especially typhoid and cholera, in addition to the overcrowding and the nonexistent hygiene of staff and patients alike, all caught her attention. Her early efforts to communicate these observations were ignored.

After witnessing these terrible wartime conditions, Nightingale returned to England to share her views with politicians back home. She communicated to British newspapers what she witnessed and the beginnings of solutions to correct the problems, promoting government interventions. She explained to anyone who would listen how hygienic conditions could alleviate unnecessary deaths. She asked for funds to build a hospital designed differently. She collected data on patients who had received care that involved simple principles of hand washing and wound care practices that caused less cross contamination between patients. She separated out causes of death to differentiate death by a bullet or bayonet versus the complications of surviving the initial injury but dying as a patient in the hospital. For the first time in history, she revealed that death rates decreased by 40 percent when the measures she put into place were followed. Based on her earlier mathematical education, she depicted these causes of deaths through "pie charts." This visual presentation of her information opened the

What impressed me the most was that Nightingale advocated that all patients had the right to better care than what they were receiving. War was unjust to its victims but Nightingale methodically envisioned care that she believed would result in less suffering and less morbidity and mortality, based solely on what she believed was within the realm of being a nurse.

minds of political and medical leaders to the magnitude and complexities of patient deaths as a result of multiple causes.

After Nightingale returned to England from the Crimean War, she continued to collect evidence on the health of the soldiers in the Royal Army, testifying exactly how the establishment of sanitary conditions had saved lives. Her information began to resonate. The U.S. government sought her advice and recommendations in the 1860s because it was now fighting its own Civil War. She developed the first School of Nursing, associated with the highly respected King's College in London, graduating its first students in 1860. Nightingale's time to be heard had come. She followed her convictions and her vision of providing care that was organized differently. She approached nursing in a professional manner never before applied to the care given by women to patients needing *nursing care.*

Nightingale advocated that all patients had the right to care that was hygienic, all of the soldiers, officers and non-ranking military men alike, which was better care than what they were currently receiving. From the battlefield she moved on to advocate for improved care for prostitutes and criminals.

Within her book, *Notes on Nursing,* Nightingale, in 139 pages, wrote about the skills and attitudes needed to care for sick or dying patients. At that time, comfort and the spread of disease were foremost on her mind. *Notes on Nursing* represented the first time that nursing care had been described as uniquely different from care delivered by physicians.

The conclusions she reached were profoundly prescient and far-reaching. Her observations regarding staff and patient hygiene, the spread of disease, and nutrition were original. She organized patients into groups so that the care they received would be more efficient for those providing the care and safer for patients. None of these concepts had been considered prior to her observations. She developed the practice of keeping infected patients separate from those with open wounds and those who had surgery. These changes were monumental and remain in place today.

She believed nurses possessed a set of skills based on provable knowledge different from that of physicians. She sought out politicians, educators, and wealthy people to extol that this knowledge and these skills were worthy of being taught in a formal academic setting to students calling themselves nurses. Good, sound nursing care did make a difference as to whether people lived or died. Nightingale worked to communicate her beliefs to decision makers; those who possessed money and influence. More than one hundred years later many of Nightingale's observations and recommendations remain.

I look to this tenacious, dedicated, steadfast figure for inspiration today and invite other male and female nurses to consider the legacy she left us. Her belief that nurses should feel called to provide care was sophisticated enough that she stated: "Patients receive the best care when no single power is ascendant. There is a perpetual rub" between those involved in the delivery of care that "often does not serve the patient." This insight remains applicable today. Nurses, physicians and other members of the health care team continue to have disagreements on who should be "in charge."

Nightingale's greatness lies in tackling what she considered the problems of her time. She both chose her battles and at the same time, responded to what needed to be done. Many of these were seemingly small battles that became crusades of hers for a lifetime. Her recommendations resulted in the reorganization of nursing tasks in hospitals all over Europe and the world by the end of her lifetime in 1910.

She was later given many accolades for her actions, though this attention never seemed important to her. She responded to her own feeling that simple things could make a difference in patients' lives. She believed that care should not be different for those patients that had money. She fought for funding to put into practice what her data indicated regarding hygiene and patient care. Her battles were not glamorous, but she put one foot in front of the other and did what she could do to make life better for patients in many environments besides hospitals.

Nurses continue to fight for patients today. The battles confronting nurses today are often not considered important, but just as in Nightingale's time, if believing that each and every patient's needs could be improved upon by your efforts, with no guarantees other than nurses each responding to their own barometer of what excellent care is, then this is admirable.

Author, Victoria Sweet, MD in *God's Hotel: A Doctor, a Hospital, and a Pilgrimage to the Heart of Medicine* that Nightingale was an "optimist, a person that stated that God wanted us to make mistakes, that mistakes are the basis of evolution." Nightingale did not shy away or give up when her concerns were ignored. She exhibited steadfast courage and tenacity when she was openly discounted by those that based their decisions not on facts, but on their own ignorance.

If we are to go on living together on this earth,
We must all be responsible for it.

—Kofi Annan, 2001 Nobel Peace Prize Winner

CHAPTER 3

A Lifetime of Firsts, Starting Right Now

What is just beyond where you are now,
what is just beyond what you cannot see?

A lot of times, people ask me, "Do you remember your first patient?"

There are so many kinds of "first patients." There is the first patient I felt I really helped, the first one I connected with on a deep level, the first time I saw a baby born, the first time I know I saved someone's life, and the first dead person I had ever seen or touched.

The very first time I was responsible for a patient, where I was someone's full-fledged nurse ... I do remember.

—GRADUATION, JUNE 1971

My classmates at Providence all were going to take two weeks, four weeks, or the rest of the summer off, but not me. I started orientation at Stanford University's intensive care unit (ICU) 30 hours after I became an RN. I was that excited! It was an amazing place to be accepted as the first new grad, with no experience, that Stanford had ever accepted to go right into its ICU. The hospital was known for its state-of-the-art equipment, medical school, and care given to patients, especially patients needing open-heart surgery.

I was well aware of how sick the ICU patients were because patients came from all over the world to find out what was wrong with them, all hoping for a cure. My orientation as a new graduate was three months long. I learned so much it made me wonder what I had learned in school! I took notes on three-by-five-inch cards and kept them in my pocket for quick reference on the science behind every vital sign that went from normal to abnormal and with so many medications that it made my head swim. Knowing what was going on with these sick patients was scarier than any "nun" experience I ever had in school.

Going through the ICU orientation was much like an extension of nursing school which was a tremendous opportunity. My rent was $195 a month and I was getting married on Thanksgiving Day to my high school sweetheart. A "meal" at McDonalds cost 30 cents and a gallon of gas was 30 cents. Having not quite emerged from student mode, it was just as if this orientation was like the final, biggest challenge of being a student. I was paid $695 a month and because I had $25 extra each month, I felt rich. Life couldn't have been better!

Still, I wasn't considered ready to care for a patient on my own. In the first six months at Stanford's ICU, I had backup from one experienced nurse after another. The tips these nurses gave me while carefully watching over me felt supportive and gave me confidence. I was most impressed with how these ICU nurses seemed to effortlessly juggle so many tasks and get them all done on time. You had to monitor the patients' vital signs, give out meds on schedule, and keep track of multiple physicians; orders that resulted in you assessing the patient and then, based on their vital signs or response to the meds they were on, decide what action to take. Physicians went on their rounds twice per shift, and with their visits came changes. It was not called "time management" then, but that's what it was.

The day arrived when I reported to work: a real nurse who would be assigned the care of a patient, or patients, just like the other 10 nurses on duty that day. I think I'm ready for this, I went off thinking, not noticing where I had parked my sand-colored 1965 Chevy Impala my parents gave me when I graduated.

> I was so excited. I have two patients!

On my first "real" morning in the ICU, I showed up for my 7:00–3:00 shift 10 minutes early, in my white fitted uniform, white cap with the stripe across the edge and my Providence College of Nursing pin that all nurses wore from the place they had received their degree. I hoped I had a look of optimism and seriousness. My excitement was contained. I didn't want anyone to worry that I wouldn't be able to carry out my responsibilities. I had pens in my pocket, and my long hair was pinned back and gathered under my cap; by now I had a lot of experience at doing it this way, so it felt attractive and professional.

Just like the other real nurses, I assembled with the rest of the staff at 7:00 a.m. sharp in the nurses break room to hear the change-of-shift report. These included bulletins such as, "Be careful because we're low on number 14 suction catheters," and "Be careful—someone heard there was a blood-borne pathogen found on a patient upstairs." Then came the lunch assignments, and I got the least popular time slot for lunch, 10:45 a.m. I wasn't surprised. Oh well, I thought, this is what I expected. I'm the new kid on the block.

After that came assignments, which I was waiting for breathlessly and eagerly. I waited to hear my name—there it was, Julie Hackett—and instead of announcing just one patient, there were two! Julie Hackett, ROOM 12, BRONSON AND WHITE.

I was so excited. "I have two patients!"

As we headed out to our rooms to relieve the night-shift nurses, every one of the other nurses gave me a pat on the back, or a "You'll do just fine" or "Call me if you need me; I'm next door to you today." These two people are getting a good nurse, I thought, as I strode purposefully to Room 12.

The night nurse inside Room 12 was just ending her shift, cleaning up odds and ends. I said "hello" to her as I entered, and she nodded politely to me and said, "You really lucked out: both of these patients are going to be discharged out of the ICU in the next couple of hours." Then there I was: alone with two strangers.

Mr. Bronson, a tall thin man, was in Bed A, and Mr. White, a white-haired fleshy man in his 50s, was in Bed B; both were holding pillows against their chests as they took deep breaths after first having had breathing treatments. All surgical patients are at risk for lung complications, and I knew that it hurt to cough, even with a pillow, which helps to splint the edges of their sternums, opened for their cardiac surgery. Walking, deep breathing, coughing and good hydration would replace the ICU breathing treatments.

"My name is Julie, and I'll be your nurse for today," I said. *I will do everything right, everything exactly right*, was the mantra inside my head as I went to wash my hands in the room sink. As I washed thoroughly with Phisohex, in my mind, I was saying to these two men, "Today, you are getting a good nurse!" Had I really said *that* out loud, I wondered?

"What are you washing your hands for?" Mr. Bronson said. "You didn't do anything to get dirty yet." The man was joking, of course, but I didn't hear it that way, I blushed.

When I was done washing my hands, I looked at my list of things to do: wound care, four or five meds for each of them, ambulate (walk them around the long hallway), and then take out one of their IVs, leaving in the other for the floor nurses to finish up their antibiotic course—and have all of this completed by 10:00 a.m., when visitors would be arriving. Suddenly it seemed like a lot to do. Mr. Bronson looked as if he was starting to doze off so I would start with Mr. White's wound care.

What I didn't know was that the charge nurse had given me the least sick patients on the unit. I had never actually taken care of any patients in orientation who were this well! In fact, these two men could have been discharged to the floor the day before, but there were no floor beds. It still hit me as pretty amazing that five days ago both of these men had entered the hospital after having heart attacks. Severe chest pain brought both of these men to the ER in panic as they responded to their heart muscle's message of *I'm not getting enough oxygen because one or more of my five coronary arteries is blocked. This is serious— drop what you are doing and get help now!*

I dried my hands on a clean, white towel. The room was quiet. Mr. Bronson was sort of looking at a book in between dozing; Mr. White was looking at me. I tried to look back at him in the most nurse-like, comforting way, but inside I was thinking, *What the heck do I do now?* Breakfast was still a ways off. It wasn't time to ambulate them, and it wasn't time yet for 8:00 a.m. meds. *Just whatever you do, till you think of what you should be doing, don't chatter, or they will know that this is your first day alone.*

"Are you new?" Mr. White, the older patient, asked. He meant, of course, new to the hospital.

"I'm new to you," I said brightly.

"I meant have you been a nurse long?" He clarified kindly.

"I graduated in the spring," I said politely, although I was devastated by the question. I didn't want to lie and I didn't want Mr. White to think that he had a nurse with no experience when I now had been on the unit for three months.

And because I was sure small talk was the least helpful thing I could do for these two men, I busied myself with reviewing again—and again—their orders from the Card X that had all of their orders, dates, and responses since they had gotten out of the operating room (OR). Their cards were so scribbled up that I wanted to make sure I didn't miss something such as their allergy status or something life threatening.

I was relieved to hear the clattering of the breakfast carts outside the room. I helped adjust the men's pillows and bed heights as they ate their morning meal. After the two men ate off their trays with surprisingly (to me) good appetites, I asked, "Who's up for wound care first?"

"How about we start on your wound care," I said to Mr. Bronson, after he had finished and put aside his tray.

"Oh, no," he answered. "I'm going to the bathroom *right now*."

That left Mr. White. Wound care consisted of cleaning the 12-inch-long mid-sternal wound and the two 24-inch leg wounds where the cardiac surgeons had taken segments of his saphenous veins to place in his heart when his blocked coronary artery was removed. When I was done, I looked around. Where was Mr. Bronson? Was he still in the bathroom? I didn't think so, but I checked. Nope. No one in the bathroom. I looked around the room with rising desperation. He was not here, and I doubted that he should be out of my eyesight.

Dashing to the door, I saw Mr. Bronson down the hall, walking along with his IV pole. "You wait here," I told a befuddled Mr. White, and ran after my patient. (By the way, that's what a nurse isn't supposed to do—leave the room and patients to which she or he is assigned.)

As I ran, I heard, "What are you doing out in the hallway, Julie?" and I turned to see the charge nurse running after me.

"He—ran out," I told her, somewhat out of breath.

"You know you're not supposed to leave the patients' rooms—that's why we assign float nurses, to get whatever you need because we have separate patient rooms in our ICU. I panicked when I saw you running. Let me find your lost patient."

I was embarrassed. Really, how was a middle-aged man, still clutching his pillow to his chest, with his rear-end showing, going to escape? I was getting frazzled. *Calm down, no one saw this silly response of yours,* I thought as I returned to find Mr. White snoozing with clean white dressings patched all over his body.

Mr. Bronson returned and looked less grumpy as he said, "I just didn't want to go to the bathroom in our room. I wanted some privacy after being with people for the last five days." We didn't talk as I expertly changed his wound dressings.

As I was finishing up with Mr. Bronson, I realized, with a sinking stomach, that I was behind on meds. How was it 9:25 a.m. already? I got them both medicated a little later than 9:00, but neither of these two gentlemen mentioned this to me.

This had never happened in orientation, and I came from a school that had plenty of clinical hours in its curriculum, so why did I feel like I had lost control or should have been better? I had been behind on meds, the charge nurse had already reprimanded me, and now their visitors would soon be arriving.

In my haste to put away any grooming, breakfast, and care items, I knocked a pill bottle off of the med area by the sink. It noisily rolled under the bed, farther and farther from my grasp. I didn't swear back then, aloud or silently; that would come later. I also didn't have any other choice than to kneel down, in the most undignified position, and pick it up. And as I was down there, I realized that I still had not done any charting as to what I had done. Of course, it was at this moment that the charge nurse came in to see if I needed any help, and because there were no orders on either patient's charts that necessitated being on the floor, she was just about to ask me AGAIN what I was doing, but then thought better of asking this question and just walked away.

"I'm so hot!" I thought. "How did it get so hot in here?" Visiting hours came suddenly, in the middle of my charting. Mr. White's family surrounded his bed, chatting. Then in walked his doctor to discharge him to the floor. As I was trying to think of some insightful comment to make, Mr. White leaned around his wife, whose hand he was holding, and said, "I've got the prettiest little nurse in the whole ICU. I must be special."

"Yes, she is," said the surgeon as he walked into the room.

Was this a compliment, or were they just being nice to a young incompetent nurse, new on the job?

Just then I realized that Mr. Bronson was gone again!

Déjà vu; what was I supposed to do? Stay in the room or leave my missing patient to fend for himself? *At least the surgeon hadn't asked where my second patient was,* as he turned to speak with Mr. and Mrs. White.

My heart pounding with all the "what-ifs," I went to search for Mr. Bronson. I found him outside, still with his IV pole, standing by a tree. He just didn't like staying put. He was "bored," he said—and wanted to "feel the sun as I realized how lucky I was to be alive." I nodded as I felt his moment of joy and understood how amazing this day was in his life. Mine, too, I wanted to say but didn't as we headed back inside.

"I saw the doctor just before I left and told him that I felt as good as new," he serenely said.

I replied, "You are as good as new. I wish the best for you." That explained why the surgeon hadn't asked where Mr. Bronson was, I now realized. He had done an *eyeball exam* of his patient and decided he looked good enough to leave the ICU. A stop outside in the sun was also OK.

I'd never taken my 10:45 lunch, so I was starving. I was exhausted, although I knew that I hadn't done anything much to feel this way. The 3:00–11:00 evening-shift nurse entered the room just as the orderlies wheeled both men to their final hospital beds, on the way to going home a few days later.

"Bye, Honey," Mr. Bronson waved. "Don't be losing any more patients today."

I smiled and left as the evening nurse prepared to receive a really sick man that hadn't done well in the OR and would require all of her attention.

"No, thanks, I won't need your help," she responded nicely when I asked her if she need any help.

Fortunately, the parking lot was almost empty. All my shift mates knew where their cars were parked and had left. Their vacated spaces helped me to see my car parked right behind where I was standing. I drove to my home in Menlo Park, feeling exhausted, but as I drove off, I could feel my mouth pulling into a grin that contained a sigh of complete contentment.

Do all that you can to preserve hope,
believe that your future will be better
than it might seem right now,
see the power that you do have
and direct it towards yourself.
Recognize that there are many paths
to one's goals, and last, know that there
will be obstacles, and you have the power
to overcome them.

—Paula Davis-Lacack, coach

CHAPTER 4

Confidence Replaced Fear: Getting the Hang of IT— One Year Later

I felt the *sacredness*—the only word that
applies here—of what went on between me,
my patient, and his wife.

*I gift you with the courage to be, to know deeply
the divine design of your life. I gift you with the
passion for the possible and the willingness to
bring this possibility into time. You are more
than you think you are and something in
you knows this.*

—JEAN HOUSTON, PhD, SCHOLAR, AUTHOR

No longer a novice but still inexperienced
after the first year, I was a different person.
I didn't worry that I might get a patient "too sick"
for me to manage. I had a healthy respect for the unpredictable
and mysterious human body, but I was no longer tense coming

from the parking lot into the hospital. This had been replaced by excitement. I had learned the answer to the question that would remain important every day of my career: what to do if you had a question about your patient—recognize what you knew and what you didn't know, and then ask; it could mean the difference between life or death to your patient.

There were so many people willing to teach you, I just had to listen to the many doctors, nurses, researchers, pharmacists, and especially to the patients. I learned to ask questions, and more importantly, I trusted myself when something didn't seem *right*. I knew that asking for validation of what might be a hunch was in the patients' best interest.

When I look back, one particular patient stands out, not because he was sicker in some outstanding way or due to anything unusual happening when I was with him. I think I remember this specific patient because it was around then that I came to know that this "sixth sense" I had been developing came from the same place in me as it did in the physicians. It could be fact based, experience based, or intuition based, but it could be trusted. This was not because anyone was *always right* but because I was right often enough that if I hadn't listened to my inner voice, then the patient could have been in danger.

I had begun taking care of the heart transplant patients, and this was an honor. Stanford did the second heart transplant in the world and continued to do about one a month the entire time I was there. Dr. Norm Shumway was an icon to all of the clinical staffs. He was warm and personable as he held the hands of patients and their spouses before and after their surgeries. He never acted as if any patient's surgery was routine. To me, this quiet man embodied what being a great doctor was.

A sales manager with a good job and a family waiting for him, Bill T. had a wide, Irish face, pale blue eyes, and a kind smile. However, he hadn't smiled for a while now. A heart transplant patient, he'd been on the operating table for a long nine hours, and as soon as he was off of the table, his recovery didn't go smoothly. Sometimes that just happened. Some patients did well with their heart surgery, and others reacted in ways no one expected. Everyone suspected this man wasn't going to make it, but even I had seen patients no one thought would make it, and they did. I was still on the hopeful side, surprised when someone didn't make it, and I was sure Bill was sick but would walk out of this place, fortunate to be alive and going home.

When I came into Bill's room his second post-op night, I thought to myself that it wasn't possible for this man to have any more medications running through four IV lines. One line was for vasodilators to open up circulation to his heart and body; one was for vasoconstrictors to keep blood shunted to the vital areas of his head, heart, and lungs; another one was for antibiotics and immunosuppressant medication to give this new alien heart a chance to make it in its new home; and one was for fluids and as a backup for meds that might be ordered and were incompatible with the meds in the other lines.

In addition to the IV lines, there was a respiratory ventilator to breathe for him until he was out of the woods and could breathe on his own, which occurred sometimes in 12 hours or sometimes not for weeks. The sooner the better was always more desirable.

An important part of interacting with a patient, I'd learned, was to say, "Tell me or show me where it hurts" when doing a particular procedure or just sitting beside someone and I sensed pain. However, with this patient, as with others in similar conditions, I had to rely on my own sense of his tolerance and comfort level, because at this point, Bill couldn't talk. His hands were loosely retrained to prevent him from trying to pull out one of his tubes, a normal response to being in pain and disoriented. He had two chest tubes in his lungs attached to two Hemovacs, bubbling plastic containers that helped keep his lungs inflated and free of any accumulating blood. He also had a fifth line that I started almost as soon as I got there, for him to receive one, then two, then five units of blood and fresh frozen plasma (FFP) to assist with what appeared to be bleeding that wouldn't stop.

I had to suction Bill often to clear out mucus accumulating in his lungs because his new heart wasn't pumping strongly enough to keep his lungs clear. His new heart had to keep itself perfused and alive first before it could work to get an optimum amount of blood to his head and lungs.

> Sometimes it's hard to find a square inch on a patient to touch that isn't going to interrupt some medical process.

Hour after hour, I adjusted his meds and IV fluids, while keeping an eye on his respiratory status. He was beginning to "lighten up" a bit. He was being weaned off the meds given to him to relax and reduce the workload on his heart. I washed Bill's face. It wasn't medically necessary, but I knew he would feel better with some of the ointment and crust over his eyes removed. I used lemon/glycerin swabs in his mouth.

His wife of 25 years had been in the room off and on between the physicians who came in every 30 to 60 minutes. She was weary, and she sensed that her Bill was causing us worry. She dozed in the waiting room, refusing offers for hospital food or juice. "Not now, in a bit," she softly replied when asked by the social workers, and then housekeeping at 4:00 a.m., and even Dr. Shumway at 6:00 a.m. when he came in to see Bill after first going over to her slumped body in the waiting room. She didn't have to ask. She knew we were all full of hope, but her husband was not going to have it easy.

Sometimes it's hard to find a square inch on a patient to touch that isn't going to interrupt some medical process. But we all have hands and feet that can be lovingly touched. Gentle strokes can translate as much as eye contact or spoken words. I reached under his blanket with his wife's hand to have her tenderly touch his feet. When she and I were alone with Bill, I continued to tell her about what was going on or to explain a word I was pretty sure was unclear. She moved up to his face and touched his mouth, his ears, his eyelids.

We both sensed his needs as the monitors were beeping, the ventilator was droning, the door opened and closed, papers were rattled as his chart was examined, and voices spoke at various places around his bedside.

I felt the *sacredness*—the only word that applies here— of what was occurring between me, my patient, and his wife. This night turned into be a 12-hour shift, but because he was in a darkened, isolated room, each hour felt timeless compared with the night-day rhythms of the outside world. *Healing is an inward journey; as much as it is an outward struggle, I was learning.*

Part of me—a small part—was in this person, not able to talk, frightened, and hurting all over. I felt connected to Bill and his wife. All of the bustling activity beyond his door in the ICU didn't matter to Bill, his wife or I. With each breath, Bill labored to stay alive, we surrounded him with our energy. Hour after hour it felt as if our hearts were all beating as one.

I left Bill's room at 11:00 the next morning. His wife was sleeping beside him in a chair with her head next to his legs. I didn't know if he would be there when I came back twelve hours later. Strangely, I felt peaceful. These twelve hours now felt like only moments. *They did not feel like work.*

Driving home, squinting from the bright sun, I realized that being with Bill and his wife was not about what lay ahead for him. I didn't know if he would live or die. All I knew was that our paths had intersected and from this point on, all tasks that I performed as his or anyone's nurse were physical avenues to who the person was inside. "Inside," where the reverence of our humanness is always a given. This is awe inspiring.

Bill did leave the ICU three months after he received his new heart. I took care of him several times during this interlude and was always struck by his acceptance that his energy was better spent not worrying but in "willing his body to heal." He knew his progress was less than what was hoped for, but he was transferred to a "step-down" unit. This was a day he did not expect to see, his wife told us.

Six months after receiving his new heart, but never having left the step-down unit, Bill passed on. *Living* in the hospital appeared to many of us a dreary existence. We would see Bill and his wife pushing his IV pole through the hallways or sitting close to each other in a semiprivate living room area designed for patients who could leave their rooms but could not go far. Via conversations later related to us, we heard that Bill and his wife did not find this life disappointing. They were grateful for the six months they had with each other. They made the most of what they were given.

What they gave all of us was the honor to care for them. What we received from being a part of their health journey was more than what we gave to them the entire time we were in each other's lives.

Without my knowing it then, Bill was a part of my journey in understanding that we don't always get the life we want, but to put energy into wishing life were better or easier, or in Bill's case healthier, would have meant not living. I felt that he *should* have lived; I felt that life had been *unfair* to this gentle man. "Patients die," he said to a nurse he was close to, and she repeated to me when she saw how sad I was the morning after he died. How they *live* is what they want to be remembered by, he had told her, and he was so right.

You must give birth to your images.
They are the future waiting to be born.
Fear not the strangeness you feel.
The future must enter you long before
it happens. Just wait for the birth,
for the hour of clarity.

—RAINER MARIA RILKE, poet, existentialist writer, 1899

CHAPTER 5

Oops, Maybe I Wasn't as Smart as I Thought I Was

What really got my attention was how every one of them was laughing, looking like they were having the best time—smoking and laughing, with a group of uniformed policemen, right under a sign that said "No Loitering."

Everyone is a story, without knowing a patient's story we are technicians in the dark.
—DAVID B. MORRIS, PhD

got my suitcase from baggage claim, my heart beating a little faster with excitement. Was coming out to Colorado an impulse decision, or was this where I was meant to be? These questions played in my mind for the umpteenth time as I walked out to wait for my friend, Barb, to pick me up. I looked up and smiled. There it was, Colorado's blue sky, which "provided Coloradans with the nation's most envied weather and views imaginable," I had just read in the United Airlines magazine. It was now the fall of 1979.

Looking at the healthy, friendly faces around me, I felt encouraged. Would this be where I could begin to navigate what being single was like? I had not been "single" since I was 15. Jim and I had been together half of our lives, up until now. Now it would be "I," not "we." Had I flown out here because I didn't want to remain living in Europe? No, it was more complicated than that. I was still in love with my soon-to-be-ex-husband, but it was a love I felt was destined to be sad. Starting over was not what I had ever planned, and as scary as it was to be alone for the first time in my life, Colorado immediately resonated with my need for a new frontier. I didn't know how to be alone or to date, but I did know what love was, and it would turn out that many people stopped for a while here in Colorado in search of a new life. Just as I was now doing after 8 years at Stanford and in Germany.

Through the nursing grapevine, I'd gotten additional info about well-known Denver General, which everyone called DG. It had a really cool emergency room (ER), and that was where I would look for a position. It was a hospital providing innovative care in the newly forming physician specialty of emergency medicine.

There she was! Barb, dark hair pulled back in a ponytail; a bright-red, checkered, flannel shirt, and tight jeans—everything but the cowgirl hat! She was driving a slightly beat-up, orange Jeep with a big trailer hitch on it (to tow what, I wondered?).

I climbed in and we started chatting, both of us interrupting each other as we caught up on where nurse friends were living now, and did I know that John, the hottest ER doctor at Stanford we both knew, was working out here at DG! "No!" I exclaimed. "That is too much!" (I think I even squealed.)

I was chattering as fast as Barb, but I was also thinking ahead to the interview I had flown out here to do. I was wearing an outfit I knew would make a great impression: a navy blue Brooks Brothers suit, a crisp white blouse, and a new pair of navy heels. While I was diving into my purse looking for my sunglasses because somehow the sun seemed *especially* bright out here, Barb smiled and stepped on the gas. Noticing her adorable cowboy boots, I had the uneasy feeling I might be overdressed.

"Don't worry about being overdressed. No one cares about that out here," she stated as if she had read my mind. Her tight jeans and plaid shirt with rolled-up sleeves surprised me a little at how "Wild West" Denver might be.

"You know, we have three hours," she said. "Why don't we go have lunch in Boulder?"

"Sure," I said, suddenly wondering if I could crawl into the backseat and change into something more casual. I wished I could peel off my nylons. They had seemed like just the perfect touch this morning when I dressed, sheer and off-white, contrasting perfectly with all the dark blue.

"You just relax," Barb told me. "Lean back and close your eyes."

I leaned back and relaxed, but I never once thought of closing my eyes. The view heading west to Boulder was rivetingly beautiful. The mountains got bigger and closer. I remembered the wonder of the Swiss Alps and thought these mountains were their equal. The majestic scenery made me speechless. The feeling of uncertainty that I had taken a chance on coming here to look for a job was eroding the doubtful side of my self-talk.

It was a good thing I was not attempting to drive because I was unprepared at how beautiful this freeway drive was as soon as we left I-25 and hit US 36. The airplane magazine made Colorado sound amazing, but it couldn't describe the perfectness of this welcome to Colorado.

Driving back to Denver didn't take long enough for me. I put on some lipstick, then let down my waist-length hair and rewound it back into a tight, stylish chignon as we got closer to the hospital. Closer was all that we could get because of slow, jaywalking people crossing the nearby neighboring streets. Where there weren't people milling around, there were late-model cars that didn't sound like they had mufflers, trolling around.

> I smiled determinedly as I entered the revolving door of the hospital—a smile wiped off my face when I was almost knocked down by Zorro.

"There are lots of cars double parked at the hospital front door," Barb remarked. "How about if I let you off and then find a space?" This seemed like a good idea because the only available, questionably legal spaces we had seen were covered in broken glass. I didn't have time to make a plan on how to find each other later. I had confidence that she'd figure it out for us.

Standing at the entrance to the ER was a group of what I took to be nurses, even though they weren't wearing the blue scrubs that were standard issue in every hospital. No, they were wearing gold-colored scrubs, but what really got my attention was how every one of them was laughing, looking like they were having the best time—smoking and laughing, with a group of uniformed policemen, right under a sign that said "No Loitering." The sign, if I wasn't mistaken, was filled with bullet-sized holes. Bullet holes!

I smiled determinedly as I entered the revolving door of the hospital—my smile vanished face when I was almost knocked down by Zorro.

A man dressed all in black, wearing a black mask that covered his eyes and most of his face, came barreling toward me. He could have been any age, his voice not a giveaway because he was screaming in Spanish. Although I didn't speak Spanish well, I would have bet money that he was shrieking obscenities. This was because of the gesticulations he was making and the looks on the faces of the people toward whom he was charging.

As he dashed past me, I noticed his mask was several sizes too large for his face. He kept pushing the slipping mask back in place, but that didn't deter him from also holding out a sword (sword?!) with his right hand. His left arm, outstretched in true warrior fashion, was pushing people out of his way.

I wondered when a doctor or nurse would take charge and do something. For a fleeting moment, I wondered if I should step in and find out from which psych floor bed this man had escaped, but my good suit and heels prevented any more thinking along those lines.

No one was staring at this man, I realized, but me. He disappeared into the crowd of people in the lobby, where his noise blended in with the shouting going on there. Everyone seemed to be talking VERY LOUDLY. Snippets of sentences ... "don't want to" ... "Get me some quick" ... "not in this shithole" ... "get outta my way," all directed at whoever took the challenge to make eye contact.

I was headed for the ER usually well marked, but not here. I looked around, hoping to see some standard hospital employees—a doctor, nurse, or receptionist—someone to point me in the right direction. My gaze then got directed to a line of prisoners coming toward me, chain-gang style.

Seeing their bright orange outfits and because they were shackled together with chains at their ankles and wrists, I guessed they were prisoners. They walked in pairs, their progress slow and noisy. Every time one of them moved, the chains clanked.

I stood rooted to the spot, my heart sinking at their misfortune and I assumed, humiliation. But none of them appeared upset. Their hands gestured in the air, clanking with emphasis, as each of them, it seemed, told a story or joke to the uniformed cop beside him or the prisoner next to him. Several of the police officers were laughing at what the prisoners had to say.

"Got a cigarette, Miss?" An older black prisoner smiled at me and asked me nicely. But before I could politely answer no, I didn't have one, a guard yanked the prisoner's chain—and then winked at me. I had no idea if I should wink back, smile, or just shrug, casual-like-because I'd seen *Cool Hand Luke* and knew all about prisoners, but that was certainly not how I felt inside. My heart was heavy with embarrassment for these men, but somehow this emotion seemed wasted. Everyone was jovial except for me.

The line shuffled past me—*clank, clank*—and the smell, a dirty, unwashed funk, wafted over me. When the prisoners were a good 50 feet away, I could still smell the unpleasant, persistent smell of body odor. I stopped looking after them because my attention was caught by a familiar, albeit unpleasant sound— flesh smacking flesh. I turned to see a young woman, hardly more than a child herself, smacking a little girl on her arm. The child, probably no more than two, was shrieking. The mother was yelling, "Shut up, you, I'll give you something to cry about when we get home unless you shut your mouth up right now!"

I realized I was on my own. Anyone I saw who looked even vaguely like hospital personnel was either busy, upset, or running somewhere. I looked around, trying not to breathe too deeply, and saw—ahh, there it was—a long red arrow next to the words "Emergency Departmen". I assumed the "t" was missing, but it was enough of a direction for me.

Walking down the corridor the red arrow seemed to indicate, I encountered more people: a group of women, mostly dark-skinned, in tiny, short skirts and low-cut tops; a baby running around with no diaper on or any discernible hospital staff. What was coming at me fast was a white-haired, bent-over woman stabbing her cane at anyone she could reach.

I stayed close to the right side of the corridor and almost ran into some young guys in scrubs—orderlies, I was sure, but they didn't act like any orderlies I'd ever seen. They were laughing uproariously and wheeling some broken-down wheelchairs with deflated rubber tires really fast. One of them took a cigarette out of the folds of his rolled-up sleeve and passed it over to a patient strolling in the opposite direction, wheeling an IV pole with two empty bags of IV fluid dangling from a bent hook.

Everything was so broken looking—so broken. It was a shithole.

The patient took the cigarette, smiling with glee while whooping it up with his other gang looking "friends." This wasn't a hospital—people didn't look sick—it was a social gathering place. A man's T-shirt said, "Come join me here and have the best time in your life" (with a Disney logo).

Everything was so broken-looking—so broken. It was a shithole, I said to myself, startled at the word that came to mind. I'd been here barely 15 minutes, and *I was already sinking down to swearing.*

Two swinging doors, with "Emergency Department" painted in red letters, opened. Where would I go even if I had contemplated not sticking around?

The nurse who greeted me, a tiny person, seemed distracted. It was obvious from her cursory glance at my *vast* resumé that I wasn't impressive. I thought I was and that gave me confidence, as she dismissed me into a small office that was piled up with stacks of papers that looked like they had been there a long time. The seat cushion of the chair was, not surprisingly, torn.

The nurse said her name was Kathy and she acknowledged I was in the right place. "I was supposed to see someone named Margo," I said helpfully. Yes, they knew I was coming, Kathy told me.

"I'll get Margo, but she's really busy," said the nurse.

I waited, perched on the edge of the chair with no idea what to make of this place. Margo, a very polished appearing nurse came in to interview me.

"You'll have a lot to learn if you work here," she said, her face impassive.

She looked at my resume again and sighed. "But we're short staffed. When do you think you could start?"

I was stunned. *When could I start? This was my interview?*

Of course I wouldn't work here, I thought to myself, but I was determined not to be thrown by anything in this conversation. "Um, in three or four weeks," I said.

"Mmmm—how 'bout in seven days?" Margo countered. She'd picked up another piece of paper (it looked like scheduling), and intently scanned it. I truly didn't think she was paying attention to me at all. Had she already added, "Smith" to it?

"Oh, sure," I joked. "In a week, that's fine."

I was being my polite self, but my mind was racing as I left her office thinking *I seriously doubt that I will ever work here. I hate to be a snob, but this place is a dump! This was supposed to be the place that was going to define a new level of innovative patient care. I find that hard to believe!*

On the way out of Margo's office, looking for the exit hallway to guide me to where I'd find some fresh air, I passed Kathy. "Hey, wait. I'm supposed to give you a tour," she said with a friendly smile. "Oh sure, great," I replied like a thief caught trying to make a run for it before someone discovers he is a con.

I really wanted to find a restroom and leave, but on second thought, I was pretty sure I could hold it. The restrooms had to look and smell as funky or worse than what my own sweat was going to smell like as it seeped from my skin through my overdressed suit. This place looked more like the place the twenty-first century would be bypassing as the *pioneering* Mecca for innovative anything, was my humble opinion.

The tour consisted of: "Here are the medicine rooms, the trauma rooms, and the jail; do you have any questions?" Kathy asked.

The *jail*, I thought, even if I was curious to see a *real* jail in an ER. I replied, "No thanks, I have a ride waiting for me." I smiled my most poised fake smile and clicked my smart navy pumps shrilly on the cracked linoleum floor.

There had been no thought in my mind of "Should I take a risk and come back, or should I just forget about my one day in Colorado?"

When I showed up ten days later, I saw Kathy's halfway grin and learned that she gave me such a quickie tour because she figured I'd be a "for sure no-show." My classy, tight smile had been the giveaway. She told me, "You can tell those nurses that are way outta their league the minute they walk into the department. I figured you to not be able to see that as crazy as this place is, and as old-appearing as it is, that there is energy here. Hell, the trauma rooms alone were set up like no other trauma rooms anywhere else if you'd really looked in the rooms when I took you by them."

I had missed the cues she was talking about, but I had felt the energy underneath everything else that had turned me off—vital, fierce energy as magnetic to me as the "Gateway to the Rocky Mountains" drive had been.

Who was the first person to tell you
that you were good at something?
You know how you felt
as you remember this moment.
Thank this person and leave this legacy
to someone else.

—BRAD MELTZER, author

CHAPTER 6

This IS My World

It was humbling, and it was scary to those of us
who were young because even though we
had seen a lot, maybe we could become people
like this if we were *unlucky*.

*In the most helpless moments of our lives,
we must truly rely upon the kindness of strangers.*
—DANIEL F. CHAMBLISS, AUTHOR

hen did I decide to stay at Denver General (DG)? It is impossible to think of an exact day or month when that happened or recall a particular event that caused me to say, "I'll stay." No. It was more like I had made a life in Colorado, and DG was at the heart of it. Gradually, I knew that this was my world.

The azure Colorado sky, stretching endlessly overhead, was now so familiar. The freedom it promised was now part of my daily life. Along with the state's other residents, I was now an avid skier, rock climber, and hiker. Hiking had become my special joy, and my favorite place to hike was the 8.5 miles up the breathtaking Conundrum Pass, near Aspen. This long day hike takes you through the Maroon Bells and through Snowmass to the most beautiful hot springs of Conundrum Peak and Castle Peak. Both "14-teeners" with gorgeous mountains on either side.

My three-week orientation at DG was the shortest orientation ever. Well, except for my orientation in the all-German-speaking open-heart surgery unit in Kiel, Germany, when I had no idea how long my orientation was because I did not speak a word of German. These nurses taught by a see-one-do-one buddy system, and they thought I didn't speak German, as the new "American schwester" because I was shy. Once again I carried 3x5 index cards in my pocket to frantically learn. The fact that I had made it in a totally all German speaking setting gave me an opportunity to see how resilient and up to a challenge I had it in me to be. I learned to speak German very well in the 18 months I worked there.

However, as it turned out, both orientations were *enough*— enough to be scared but in high alert mode, knowing it would be up to me to figure out fast what to do and to whom to turn to if I really needed a question answered. I took my cues from the other staff. They didn't act like they thought DG was out of control; in fact, they seemed to relish all the noise and the challenge of searching for the equipment they needed. No one, docs or nurses, asked anyone to get the stuff he or she needed. You went and found what you wanted and didn't go through a pecking order of finding someone in a lower position to procure it. This was a first, and though I didn't understand it at first, I liked it.

My life in Colorado was richer than I'd imagined; my colleagues were fast becoming good, dear friends. It wasn't just the nurses; a large group of people were part of the ER landscape. Firefighters and cops dropped off patients whose heart attacks or four-day drinking binges they'd intercepted. These guys

appeared so often they felt like part of our team; they certainly
became familiar and in some cases "significant others." Romances
occurred often because of our similar hours and the "war stories"
that we shared.

Paramedics were also part of our group. They rushed to the
scene, provided life-saving care, and then brought patients into
the ER. It was not unusual for them to stick around and help us
calm an unruly patient or to growl one last time to a patient:
"With this nurse you'd better not pull any of that shit you did
with us in the ambulance ride over here, or you'll hear from me
again, Bud." Many of the paramedics had taken the job because
they weren't sure what they wanted to do in life, and one of
these was Bruce Adams, a guy who would become a lifelong
friend of mine. We liked talking and laughing together. So many
of the paramedics, cops, and firefighters were, along with us,
young and single, and we often remarked that all of our jobs
were *young-people jobs.* They took a lot of energy and were a
lot of fun when young but would be tough after you got to be
"older, like in your 40s!"

All of us worked hard under stressful circumstances, and we
understood each other's need to relax. After each shift, we talked
about everything we'd seen and still felt the need to "process."
We often laughed at some of the more bizarre patients and events
we'd encountered, but it didn't feel condescending or mean. It
was a way to decompress from life's hardships. It often felt unfair
and seemed incomprehensible that family members, friends, or
even strangers inflicted so much hurt on each other.

We talked about neglect that became abuse, about not having
enough money to buy an over-the-counter (OTC) medicine for
your child's fever, or the choice to buy drugs and alcohol instead
of a night's shelter. How much of this was choice versus circumstances? Our real-life specifics often turned to esoteric, existential

grasping at explanations of why or how lives took such diverse doglegs. The hours meant that we sought out places like the 404 Club on Broadway, which served cocktails with breakfast, before going home to sleep.

One thing that struck me early on was how Lulu, who could be tough on some nurses, would never let anyone disrespect a patient. What I'd noticed, as well, was that different nurses, in their different ways, were empathetic and compassionate to patients, but I know that it might not have looked like this to an "outsider."

During that first walk through the hospital on the way to my interview, I remember being so horrified. Now, those same patients I'd first viewed from am alarmed distance were my reality. Some of them I was getting to know quite well because they appeared so often: DG, chaotic and noisy and smelly, was the safest place for some of these individuals.

I'm thinking in particular of Delubina, a lady in her 50s, not attractive, who seemed perpetually drunk. In Denver, intoxication is considered a medical condition, not an automatic crime. Denver was one of the first cities to establish a city-operated service that swept through all of the alleys, parks, and unlit street-corner areas with a specially trained staff looking for intoxicated people. Bars called Herb's Hideout and El Gato Negro were sites that sometimes hourly produced vulnerable folks taken to DG for treatment instead of to jail.

We understood these "tough customers." The Denver Cares van was a job that took a special type of person to troll streets picking up many times the same individuals several times a week for years and delivering them to detox centers such as Arapahoe House or Denver's Detox Center, where they could sleep it off (SIO) safely. Delubina was often in the group the police brought to the ER because she was prone to withdrawal seizures. It became obvious she might be about to seize when she became rowdy. "The van" was called for her by businesses that didn't need her troublemaking *again.*

It was our job to do a thorough exam of anyone brought into the ER. No matter how many times he or she came in, it was our responsibility to make sure the person was not in any physical danger. So when Delubina showed up, we knew she would "Honey-Baby-Sweetie Pie" you till she then turned on you with the foulest words. After spewing all manner of expletives, she would smile up at you and conk out, unless you grabbed her by whatever clothing she had on and took her to a bed in the back hallway. What I'd come to realize is that you get used to almost anything.

Then there was Cindy S., a lady for whom I felt a great deal of sympathy for the entire time I worked in the ER because she never got rescued or escaped the life by which we knew her so well. She was white and married to an abusive Hispanic man who regularly pimped her out. Cindy herself was an alcoholic, and the seizures she suffered along with the dubious state of her

> For so many of our patients, the idea of "hope" was a lost or never-realized concept.

brain because of her drinking were the worst possible combination. She often came in wearing no clothing, at least from the waist down. Cindy S. was brought in with a sheet wrapped around her that she fought with us to keep her covered until we could take her to a room to be examined and also to SIO. She had been offered detox, Social Services assistance, and police protection many times, but somehow nothing worked. We blamed her, we blamed ourselves, we blamed politicians, and some blamed a God that *should* be protecting her from herself.

It was hard to get used to the repetitive nature of these visits. When I later oriented new nurses, I told them that what helped me if I felt angry at a patient or at an entire night of patients, was to select one drunken person and ask what he or she did before booze took a hold of them. At first it surprised me when they said they were office managers, bank tellers, or other occupations that required responsibility or discipline to perform their tasks. When I asked, "What happened?" they told a story that became all too familiar: "I lost my job, had some car debt or medical debt, I drank, my wife left me, and here I am"— a course these once responsible people never imagined would have ended with their being homeless and invisible. I realized that no one grew up and said, "I want to be a drunk, pass out, have someone beat me up for a buck in my pocket, vomit on myself, piss on myself, and be treated like a worthless piece of shit."

I realized that this path could happen to anyone, to any of us staff members as well. It was humbling, and it was scary to those of us who were young because even though we had seen a lot, maybe we could become people like this if we were *unlucky*.

For so many of our patients, the idea of "hope" was a lost or never-realized concept. Some folks did seek help for their alcoholism or drug addiction, but these services provided so little of what we knew was needed to walk away from the allure of the substances and the life circumstances that could not be easily fixed.

I was never sure of what percentage of our patients were under the influence of drugs or alcohol, but we often remarked that 60 percent of our patients (more or less depending on the time of day) came in "altered." We had posters in the hall advertising the twelve-step program, but they got filled in with graffiti till eventually someone always pulled them down. It seemed to me that the extreme poverty, run-ins with the "law," and family life occurrences that stretched love beyond its limits pushed our patients to find some way to *medicate* their feelings away.

This same environment, in which teenagers did drugs and had babies, was responsible (it seemed to me) for most of the accidents that brought little kids into the ER. I remember a little girl named Rosa who came in looking stunned, with a huge goose egg on her head, having climbed on top of the kitchen table and fallen off. Where were her parents, we asked, when Rosa was climbing on top of a table? Not home, was the answer. The father was rarely home, and the mother had gone out to the store.

Then there was a four year old who stumbled down the hallway with his father, uncle, or some man who didn't know that little boys could not take long, fast steps when they had a runny nose, a cough, and wheezing that sounded like it had been present for a long time. Trying not to cry added to his misery as the older male looked much more annoyed at being in the ER than worried that the "kid is sick." Sometimes being nonjudgmental came easier than other times. This was not one of those times.

Then there were the bittersweet moments: kids having kids, children coming into the ER at the last minute, moments away from being moms for life, delivering their baby, then asking for a cigarette and being unhappy that they got a boy "when I always wanted a girl!"

Most of our patients had heard of but had not had time for finding, planning to go, or going to get prenatal care. Were they unhappy, surprised, or clueless now that the pain of labor was over? Waiting till someone else told them what was happening next only meant that this Friday night was not going to be as fun as most Friday nights were.

A memorable night would later become a picture in Eugene Richards' book *The Knife and Gun Club*. By chance he captured a night that ushered in life and death moments apart in time and space. A woman rushed in and immediately delivered her baby boy in a room that still had the body of a man who had died of a cardiac arrest. He was a homeless person, and paramedics brought him in while performing CPR after he was "found down." The laboring woman and her family—consisting of her husband, sister, and cousin—rushed in just as a sheet was placed over the man's body. In their excitement and total enchantment with their new family member, they never noticed the clear outline of death under a plain, white sheet only six feet away, on a gurney pushed against the wall. We turned off the overhead light and put on only the high-intensity surgical light, causing a dim, almost gentle look to the room as she delivered the placenta, and we then moved them to the room next door where they continued to shower love onto their new, wanted little son or cousin.

Dying and the welcoming in of new life often "collide" in hospitals. The proximity of these two events at first made me uncomfortable. Over time I felt a sense of honor and peace at being present to these events that hopefully were important in someone else's life.

Occasionally I found myself questioning if we made a difference. A judge once told me when I had to appear in court to testify as part of the chain of evidence because I had drawn blood to test for alcohol and drugs in the ER after a DUI had caused the death of a pedestrian. "You have to believe that you make a difference, even if its taken us a while to finally lock this person up. You are part of keeping our community safer."

Just as Florence Nightingale had gotten used to death on the battlefields of Crimea, I had shifted from feeling over-whelmed or insignificant to knowing that my skills had grown from being a "novice" to "expert." From life saving actions to fighting to keep a naked patient covered—it was all important.

At other hospitals, there was always a clean, white pad or paper sitting just where you could find it if you wanted to write something down, say a personal reminder to give a medication or a doctor's order. However, at DG I don't think I ever saw a piece of paper to write something down on. We used a Kleenex box or a sterile four-by-four-inch dressing wrapper, or our hands—but somehow as annoying or comical as this could be—the important stuff all did get done. We worked with the resources we had and without the ones we didn't.

Race = Class = Power
Every patient's health coverage is now
the third patient in the exam room.
Health disparities are a by-product
of social and economic disparities that exist,
for which each of us within our own "systems"
are morally obligated to not be powerless.

—Winston F. Fong, MD

PART II

THE STORIES

"Every nurse has great stories— ones that reveal pain, sorrow and unexpected joy."

Storytelling is a tradition that believes that the story speaks to the soul not to the ego. In today's world we yearn to understand, to conquer our minds, but it is not in the mind that a mythic story dwells.
—DONNA JACOB STIFE

CHAPTER 7

The Waiting Room

A cardinal rule of working here, where patients
are unwashed and odiferous, is knowing that
no one grows up wanting to lead this kind of life.

*There may or may not be a disease process
when a patient comes in to be seen, but there is
always a story. The most important story may not
be the one that you hear, more likely, it is what
is unspoken—all we do know is that medical facts
alone, are not the whole story.*
—WILLIAM JAMES, MD

Who comes to an emergency room (ER) because they want to? It is a haven and a place that saves lives, but no one wants to be in the position to need to come. A particular paramedic would state under his breath as he brought in patients to whose aid he had been called because they used the magic phrase, "I have chest pain; it feels like an elephant is sitting on my chest," (knowing that need and want are often under the complete control of the patient). "Patients do what they gotta do to get the care they need or want."

In Europe, emergency departments are known as the sites where care is delivered for "accidents and injuries"—so genteel. In the United States, the ER is regarded as the place where you hope to be "saved" if you are having a heart attack, get in a bad traffic accident, or are the victim of violence. Many large and medium-sized cities often designate one particular hospital as the site where victims without life resources (friends and family), cash, or insurance can get all of the care they need. There wasn't a lot of competition for resourseless victims of violent trauma requiring expensive and often long term hospitalizations. County hospitals filled this void and provided an excellent environment for the specialty of emergency medicine to be developed.

Instead of a family doctor, our patients who streamed into the Denver General ER lacked many things I had always thought of as normal or essential. In the winter, some didn't have gloves, a hat, or a warm coat. The children were often dressed in mismatched outfits that didn't suit the season. Mothers often didn't carry extra diapers, formula or snacks.

They almost never were driven to the ER in a car. They more likely came accompanied by a group of grandmas, sisters, and cousins all traveling by bus. If they'd arrived by car, that vehicle was generally unavailable or not working by the time the patient was ready to go home.

In the ER many of our patients were Spanish-speaking only (SSO). Even though many of these patients had loving, responsible, close-knit families and friendships, they needed help with some aspect of their lives that resulted in them coming to the ER. Whether it was language translation, bus fare, help with a child who had trouble with the law, understanding the meaning of a laboratory test result, or what to do with a "life pain or a health pain."

In short, most of our patients were living on the edge. When we offered apple juice or crackers to the children or a diaper and formula to a mother, we were met with grateful smiles.

The hospital itself suffered from certain kinds of shortages. Comfort items and hospital gowns were always in short supply. Sheets that actually covered the bed were rare items, but we did have top-notch ER Docs's, anesthesiologists, and the capability 24 hours a day to take someone in to receive life-saving surgery. Designated as *the* hospital to go to any time of the day or night, DG was officially known as a Level 1 trauma site. DG earned the reputation of being the Level 1 trauma site that could be counted on to "save lives."

In 1979, when I began working at DG's ER, the waiting room was small because most patients arrived by ambulance. Ambulances dropped their patients off at the back loading dock, a bleak-appearing place as unappealing as it sounded.

The waiting room, down a long hallway with no signs pointing to it, could be difficult to find. All patients in the early years had to walk through the patient care areas to get to the front desk, sign in, and then go to the waiting room until they were called in to be seen. By having all patients come into the ER, we were able to do a face-to-face triage (assessment of their requested reason to be seen in conjunction with our brief assessment of their health/illness/injury status). This revealed to us how critical they were which translated to the all-important order in which they would be seen.

No one wants to wait in an ER waiting room. As new patients who arrived on foot were triaged and signed in, they could hear and witness scenes that caused many of them to say, "Jesus, I thought I had it bad, but I think I'll come back later because I'm never gonna be seen, looking at all of these other people."

In ERs where the bed capacity is always less than the number of patients wishing to be seen (which is to say, almost every inner-city ER), the place one occupies on the ever-changing list the triage nurse is carrying around can result in the frustrating reality that your place on the list may not seem like you're ever going to make any forward progress. You might be right. For patients who ask why other people who came into the waiting room after them but are seen before them are told, "Because they are sicker," this is disheartening.

We told patients they would be seen in the order they signed in, and that was technically correct, but on a hot summer night on any weekend, coming back later was often a better option if they could wait. If the number of gunshot wounds or stabbings or violent accidents was high, then a patient with just ordinary (but uncomfortable) stomach pains might have to sit and wait for three, four, or even five hours.

Yes, we tried to be sensitive to each and every patient. Often we tried to squeeze in patients who had simpler health concerns, but it seemed as soon as we tried to put that kind motive into effect, we had to "bump" them back to the waiting room. Someone had come in with a more serious condition, so he or she took precedence. Walking back into the waiting room was frustrating and very often eye-opening.

The curtains separating the ER cubicles fell several feet short of the floor, and they didn't cover the side-to-side width of the cubicle leading to the busy hallway. Passing through the hallway to get to the waiting room was often an eye-opening experience because people in various stages of undress made it difficult to find a place to even avert your eyes or your children's eyes. These cubicles were bare-bones Spartan, but they had what it took to save lives.

Still, this lack of visual privacy made all of us uncomfortable knowing that the people on either side of your cubical could also hear every verbal exchange. Nurses asked patients, "So when did you last have sex? What do you use for birth control? How much vaginal bleeding are you having?" or "I won't tell your mother that you think you are pregnant, but we will talk after we get the results of your urine pregnancy test back." These pieces of intimate conversations were often not as distressing as the sounds of arguing, crying, blaming, smacking of children or spouses, or the bodily sounds we all wished to keep private but were greater than the spaces provided for this to be possible.

I'm sure everyone wondered what had made THAT big dark stain?

It was not unusual for someone in a substance-altered state to answer a question someone in the next cubical was asked loudly of a deaf older parent, thinking he or she was being asked. People would roar back, "I ain't talking to you" or "Shut up" or ask the person being verbally assaulted, "Hey, lady, you want me to come over and beat the shit out of that asshole husband of yours?" People also helped each other with offers of a spare dollar or a phone call to a worried person waiting at home who did not know they were willingly or unwillingly in the ER.

I knew—and I saw—that every part of the hospital was cleaned daily, swabbed down with disinfectant. I'd seen housekeeping staff mopping the floor in our waiting room several times a day, but it did astonish me how it never looked or seemed clean. The walls were painted an off-white that, even though I knew the room had just been painted recently, certainly never looked new (unless the paint color was called "old yellow"). The floor was covered with stained, faded linoleum of brown and yellow squares, forming a dismal checkerboard. Some "replaced" new squares sat alongside older squares, but the stains were spread out over both with no discrimination. Staring at the floors, I'm sure everyone wondered *what had made THAT big dark stain.*

Yes, someone swabbed this floor every night, and a few times during the day, with a disinfecting potion that smelled like bubble gum, but that changed the smell in the room only temporarily. There was a ventilation system operating constantly, but there was always a pervasive smell—in winter wet wool and in summer, sweat. The season-specific, funky smells were different than the always-present smells of poop, urine, blood, a wound leaking pus, and the intense body odor that came from being scared. Many of the staff members smoked, and for the first time, I understood why. Cigarettes offered their own olfactory buffer.

We nurses used to rate these smells in order of severity. The worst by far was what we called the "toxic-sock syndrome." Nothing like your old, forgotten sock left on the floor of your closet, a sock that wouldn't come off of your foot without taking significant amounts of flaky skin with it (or, in some cases, taking raw, open exudates from an open wound because the sock had worn its way into your body, having been there for so long).

Vomit mixed with blood came in a close second. Then, infected wounds, unwashed bodies, and bad breath, not like your everyday halitosis but breath that made you wonder, "How in the Lord's name could a smell like that come from someone's mouth?" This was the sort of bad breath that made anyone, no matter their political persuasion, decide to vote for universal dental care, a smell so bad it caused other patients to pick up their chairs and move them across the room.

Because our blue plastic chairs weren't bolted down, they got moved around all the time. In addition to trying to get away from an offensive smell, patients had many other reasons for shifting their seating arrangements. They wanted to sit in a family group, or they wanted to get closer to someone—or farther away. If a waiting patient had a horrible cough or gaping wound, the people near him or her would often turn their chairs around if there was only standing room available and no place to drag them elsewhere.

Bleeding comes from many places, and some sites were scarier or more offensive than others. Patients might have had large gashes on their arms or chests, but if they attempted to make bandages to cover the wounds, even if they consisted of wadded up Kleenex, then the overall feeling in the waiting room was, "This is tolerable; I can sit next to him." However, if they had uncovered wounds—on their arms, say—and especially ragged lacerations, that they were trying to control the flow of blood, but they had blood that flowed from their body onto the floor, this intruded into most peoples comfort zone. That's when the chairs were dragged to the other side of the room.

As the day went on into evening and night, the waiting room got more crowded, with no chairs or even standing space within earshot of the intercom system. This caused patients to take more drastic measures than moving their chairs around. I have come out to the waiting room to see chairs turned upside down and some individuals huddled under their chairs. Something was intolerable—the noise level, another patient getting too close—and the only way they had of getting away from it all was under their chair.

This game of musical chairs added to the confusion that already existed in the waiting room. There was a certain noise level all staff members got used to. It was as if there were roles to be doled out, and as people entered the waiting room, someone accepted a well-established *patient-in-waiting* behavior relinquished when someone else had been called in to be seen. A few just sat quietly, with no need to connect and share any aspects of their lives. The quiet people seemed to "invite" the more gregarious patients to come closer. Many in the waiting room lived lives with little privacy, so that their wants, needs, or issues with the unfairness of life spewed out nonstop.

However, this wasn't the only type of verbal patient. Chatty though they might be, many caring and helpful folks often passed through. They might stand up and tell a passing nurse, "This lady next to me, she's in bad shape, you gotta see her." Sometimes they actually knew each other, from panhandling on the same corner or living in the same homeless shelter. Catching up on gossip and news and listening to a *friend's* recital of what had gone wrong or been done to them, was often interrupted by, "Hell you think you've got it bad... ."

We also saw strangers who shared. Whatever little money these generous-in-spirit individuals had, they offered some of what they had in their pockets to someone who looked like he or she needed it more. The number of people in the waiting room acquainted with each other already at first surprised me. Then I realized that so many members of this population who had so little recognized the same look in others—the shared look of poverty. They realized everyone needed a helping hand at some time in his or her life.

The generosity of the patients, families, and friends of our patients was displayed in front of me many, many times, and it always impressed me. It was something I hadn't seen a lot of in my own, more privileged world. A patient who clearly lived on the streets would offer another a dollar to get a soda. Another patient would offer to share his room that night with someone he'd just met in the waiting room, who had or had not actually said he was homeless for the night but looked like he might be.

I overheard one woman say to another, "Here's something, Honey, you go get yourself a burger and fries—there's a McDonald's across the street," and I knew they had just met. It was, I sensed, a sort of socioeconomic club that coalesced without judgment, connecting people who had nothing except the sense they were there for each other in a world that clearly wasn't.

It was a side of human nature that never failed to validate my feeling that despite all of the violence and abusive pain and injury we saw, people were good to each other. Observing their generosity to each other was a gift to me. Many times this help, this pleasantry, or this offer of a sandwich by a fellow patient communicated that *the world does care about you; you are not invisible.* The response to suffering, from someone possibly in more pain; a stranger that might have seemed to have much less to give *from,* invoked a new level of awareness, of inspiration that came solely from patients and did not involve us, their caregivers.

Sometimes two people *connected* while waiting for care in the waiting room. We'd all see a young man start talking to a woman, and before long, they were engaged in an intense conversation— their chairs moved closer, their heads touching. That any relationship could begin in the waiting room and be sustained for too long after the initial need to give or to receive had come to an end seemly unlikely but possible. The pheromone of desperation created a human and at times sexual tension activated by distress and the risky hope that a stranger just might be able to provide.

People who were already uncomfortable, if not in real pain, had to sit up for hours or stand for hours, caring for their young, hungry, exhausted children that they had to bring with them because there was no one else to help them out with childcare.

Added to this was a sense of being on high alert because no one wanted to miss hearing his or her name being called and wait another three hours.

There was another contributor to the tension in the waiting room. Some of the people needing care were vulnerable to being asked how they *got that injury*—because no one really expected that we wouldn't recognize a stab wound or a gunshot wound. Some might have been in the country illegally and believed that maybe the doctor or nurse might give their name to authorities. Life would then get significantly harder. Fear and the need to dash out of this brief safety haven might be a condition someone had lived with a long time. *Just not tonight* seemed to be on everyone's face who tried to blend in. Fear and hope are feelings most of us probably have to experience to really appreciate this level of tension. Being afraid in this way often led a patient to give less than clear answers to the questions we posed (who did this, did they have a gun, etc.).

So many waited till their concern became what they thought of as "life threatening." Chest pain that might have indicated a pre-heart attack was now a full-blown one. Not getting prenatal care, and rather waiting till the baby is just about to be delivered often occurs as well in this vulnerable population.

The patients streamed in. On a typical day, I would see bad cases of flu, car accident victims, gunshot wounds, cardiac arrests, stab wounds, bruises, and broken bones. I'd see kids who had fallen out of windows, kids with high temperatures, kids who had been sick for weeks, and over and over, the people who had consumed too much alcohol.

We saw so many women who manifested the aftereffects of fighting with their boyfriends and husbands that even though I intellectually understood that poverty and substance abuse and

its effect on interpersonal relationships escalated outcomes to
life's minor occurrences to proportions that would take more
time, energy, assistance, and money than had initially contributed to the beginning of this cycle of destitution. I wasn't sure
yet if the "rich get richer," but I was sure that the "poor just get
poorer."

In my personal life I'd thought of a miscarriage or an
abortion as a major life event worthy of tears. Almost every night
in this ER I saw life disappearing in the form of miscarriages or
violence inflicted by women on themselves or by someone else to
end an unwanted pregnancy. No matter why, how or how often
we witnessed this event, there was pain.

One winter night a woman who couldn't have been any older
than I was—in her mid- or late 20s—came in stoically alone. No
one seemed to be with her. The chair next to her was empty. The
woman's skin was smooth and light brown, and I saw that she
was pretty, with big dark eyes and a pretty but sadly held mouth.
The prettiness of her face was marred though: her lips were
quivering, and she was banged up. There were bruises on her
face, neck, and arms. Some of those areas were an angry, deep-
red swelling.

Her clothes—a white blouse patterned with pink strawberries,
a tan jumper, maybe a maternity dress? —looked like at some
earlier time they'd been selected with care. Had she come in
without a coat?

It was not her clothing that I or anyone else who discreetly
looked at her and then me as I entered the waiting room observed,
in relief that someone had come out to talk with her. It was her
face that told of circumstances no doubt familiar to some of the
other women in the waiting room. She might have been sitting
alone, but this group of young, middle-aged, and older people

had "circled the wagons" around her, I felt. Had a man entered with her and had he been aggressive toward her, someone would have come forward, I have no doubt.

The woman had a jagged, partially congealed-red gash on her forehead, with swelling around it three times the size of the opening of her wound. She had another bruise on the side of her face that was not the same intensity, or probable age based on the color of her forehead injury. I then saw red marks on her wrists and neck. Fight markings.

After I saw these additional marks on her body, I did what I always do—assess all of the parts of her body I could see with her sitting patiently in the safety of a protective chair. She was out in the open where the light and business of other people must have been better than a dark, hidden place where she had come in from. I saw yellow-green bruises—older areas assaulted with fists or an object? Healing bruises led me to look to see if she was holding herself up with effort, if her shoulder was drooping, and if she did in fact also have on shoes that did not match. Who had come forward to sign her in, I wondered; how had she been able to walk down the hall to sign in, then walk back to the waiting room without someone stopping her to be sure that all of her injuries were even visible?

It was clear to me that this young girl was the victim of assault(s). It looked like the assault had occurred over time. As I was visualizing how crowded it was up front, I saw that there was blood on her skirt distinctly outlining her body as she remained sitting quietly but gently knotting up her hands as she held onto her stomach.

I went to crouch down beside her so that we could try to exchange a little more information without being heard and asked, "Things don't look too good with you right now?"

"I want to know if I lost my baby," she said, without looking at me. Her hands were clasped protectively around her stomach.

"What hurts the most right now?" I asked gently. "I see you are bleeding."

The young girl nodded. "He was drunk," she sobbed, "but that don't make no difference. I told him and told him, be careful of the baby, but he punched me in the stomach."

"Did the bleeding start after that?" I asked.

"Yes," she said softly.

"Let's step around the corner and go talk," I said, raising my voice above the hubbub so she could hear me.

"I can't get up because there's all this blood," she said.

"Do you have a pad on?" I asked.

"No, I used all the pads I had at home. Now I'm here," she said.

I understood that no one wants to get up and drip blood across the room. Meanwhile there are people all around, and even though I tried to talk softly, I had to speak up so this girl could hear me.

"What's your name?" I asked.

"Yolanda," she said.

"Okay, Yolanda, I'm going to go back and get something so you can walk back with me."

I went back into the ER to get a sheet. I came back to Yolanda and wrapped it around her. She was whimpering now and clutching her stomach harder.

"Is the cramping worse?" I asked, and she nodded.

If someone is bleeding and cramping with this type of history, she is likely at risk of, or in the process of, having a miscarriage.

"How pregnant do you think you are?" I asked. "Maybe three months," she responded. I told her, "Your body is doing what it's going to do right now, and we might not be able to stop what is happening. We'll get you back so that we can check you out." I could see that this young girl wanted to keep her baby, but the person I had to care about first was Yolanda; what other injuries did she have that might be serious, I wondered?

Usually, a young girl miscarrying is often not unhappy, but Yolanda seemed to be distraught that she was not able to do something to protect her baby.

I bent down to hear what she then said more to herself than to me: "I was so glad when I knew I was pregnant," she said. "Because I was going to give my little girl a different life. I was going to send her to a good school and have her be smart and not work at a McDonald's like me. She was going to have a great life, and there'd be a nice man to love her. She wouldn't have to love some mean man from the streets like I did because she'd meet a nicer man." I stood up as she asked, "Isn't that crazy?" she said. "I had it all planned out for her, and I was only three months pregnant."

Yolanda needed a friend, an aunt, another woman to be with her. "Who can I call right now to be with you?"

"I don't have nobody. I'm here all by myself." Yolanda shook her head and began to sob. As she looked for a tissue, an older black woman two seats away spoke up. "Baby, it's okay," she said, in that inimitable voice older black women have when they are comforting someone. "It's okay. I can be here with you."

The older woman had lumbered to her feet. I indicated the seat next to Yolanda, and the older woman sank down and took Yolanda in her arms. I was surprised that I had not heard my name paged overhead but knew that Yolanda could not get in to find a bed to lie on till we got someone discharged. I gave the older woman a grateful glance, jumped up, and said, "We'll hurry and find a place for you, Sweetie."

The belief that we are our brother's keeper is innate to most people's value systems. This thought connected to what Kathy told all new nurses: a cardinal rule of working here, where patients are unwashed and odiferous, is knowing that no one grows up wanting to lead this kind of life. No one grows up with the goal of becoming alcoholic or of being a pregnant woman who loses her baby because her man beats her up.

I went to put Yolanda farther ahead in line. When I came back, I didn't see her. I did see the older black woman, and I went over to her. "Where is that young girl you were comforting?" I asked. "Where's Yolanda?"

"Honey, I tried to get her to stay, but even with all that bleeding, she just up and walked out the door."

The reason I remember this particular patient was not just because I worried about what would happen to her. I had seen the stubborn light in her eyes: in all likelihood, Yolanda would be okay. She would abort this fetus in the toilet when she went home, and she would probably even hold onto her dreams. The reason I remembered her was her extraordinary dignity, and the fact that she just walked so suddenly out into the night. Regrets, sadness, and anger would propel her not to live in fear of this man, of this episode in her life.

There were and are many people that float back into my awareness that I wish I could know what had happened to them. Was life ever better or fairer to them?.

I often "completed" patients' stories when they left, and I didn't really know what happened to them. Illusions only? Self-protection from worry, guilt, and the inability to do more? Feeling powerless over the unfairness of destinies? Yes, but some of our patients had more resilience, more inner fortitude, and more hope than others. Despite life being as bad as it was when our lives intersected, I often thought that some of them would be able to rise up and not succumb to the tough events in their lives. Author Alexandra Bracken writes, "Part of surviving is being able to move on."

Our patients survived because that's what you do. *You never know how strong you are until being strong is all you can be,* is a quote attributed to many people. Finding personal strength at times that seem hopeless is a personal characteristic that always impressed me. It would later lead me to understanding the concept of nobility in nursing.

I've learned that there is no such thing
as an accident, and people make decisions
that have consequences every day.
But I don't know whether to blame the people,
the environment or genes or policy or poverty.

—Cory Siebbe, MD, Emergency Medicine

CHAPTER 8

Put on Your Virtual Glasses

No one wanted to climb up there
(although we tried to convince one young,
cute paramedic to lighten his weight by
removing his clothing and do his civic duty
by climbing up and rescuing this
maiden in distress).

Rule one of reading other people's stories is that
whenever you say 'well, that's not convincing'
the author tells you that's the bit that wasn't
made up. This is because real life is under
no obligation to be convincing.
—NEIL GAIMAN

*O*ne reason we had acronyms for everything
in the ER was because speech, like actions and
assessments, had to be done in a big hurry. After a
patient was treated, we spoke of getting him or her OTD (out
the door). When patients' actions didn't make much sense,
we put them on a MHH (mental health hold) to determine if

they'd suffered a psychotic break or some other form of mental illness. If a patient was too drunk to be walking around in the world, our doctors had the choice to place patients on what we called an "EHH," an Ethanol Health Hold (ethanol health hold). I'd been working at DG for eight years now. The acronyms seemed like second nature. So was what I called my ER nurse radar. You need the objective facts, and you need the information the paramedics give you as they rush in, but sometimes there was something inside that told me there was more to a particular patient than the initial presentation.

Funny, though: my radar didn't click in with Miss M., one of my funniest ever patient experiences, but maybe that's because she wasn't dangerous so much as inexplicable.

Miss M was brought in by the police on a busy weekend night shift. She was a large, beautiful, Hawaiian appearing woman. After getting a quick report that she "just appeared drunk," My attention was diverted to a man trying to cut in front of other patients waiting to be seen at the nearby triage desk.

"You c--t, get over here right now, I pay your salary with my taxes and I could die here waiting for some help from you."

His rant had two things that female healthcare workers hate, this particular word and being told that someone believes that their taxes or their $5.00 co-pay anywhere near pays for the care that they receive.

If there was ever a time I would have *wished* for some levity, it would be now, but that never happens! The police took care of the man at the front desk and I returned to the young woman, who was being led back to a room with the paperwork and physical restraints needed for the EHH.

Cooperative, chatty and singing. This kind of intoxicated patient can make you smile and feel that were she sober, she would be grateful that she had been taken to a safe place. Sashaying her hips and waving her arms in sexy motions as she sang out a tune I didn't recognize but that had a good beat.

The ankle strap was not prohibiting her from enjoying her dancing. Looking at her, I couldn't help smiling; she was in her own world, and it wasn't an unhappy one. I tried to pronounce her name—it began with "M.," but there were too many strange vowels in there and too many syllables for me to do it justice. I noticed that she was about 220 pounds, about five feet eight inches tall, and well dressed—which is to say her clothes were clean and appropriate to the season. Though her outfit was skimpy, she did have on underwear—always a good thing if your arms are strapped down and you can't quite reach your skirt to cover your undies. She was not fighting the one leg cuff. She didn't seem angry. She was more entertained by the shackles than steamed up about them.

"Hi, I'm Julie," I introduced myself.

The woman just kept smiling, singing, and gyrating horizontally.

"I'll be back in a few minutes," I said softly, and closed her door.

By then, I was familiar with all the stages of drunkenness. This young woman was in one of the calmer stages—happy and oblivious but not a danger to herself or others. In this stage, we know that the patients will almost certainly not vomit or aspirate their food.

Considering all of the above I thought, *She'll probably just lie there for awhile. I'd better go check on that nasty man and then in 15 minutes, I'll come back and check on my singing chick.*

Miss M. had been placed in Room 23, the last room in the medicine hallway, right next to the jail cells. This is where we usually placed patients who needed to be seen medically and were under arrest, dangerous or out of control. Miss M. did not fit the profile of this room but she was so "obtunded" (in a dreamy state because of drugs or alcohol) that this place would be a safe place to lie down until she could tell us what she had eaten or drunken earlier in the evening.

"Thanks for the singing chick," one of the deputies called out.

"Enjoy," I called back as I trotted back to the triage area.

Over the next two hours I checked on Miss M., fulfilling the legal requirements that someone on an Ethanol Health Hold must be assessed for, and recorded her signs, level of consciousness, status of the restraints to her limbs, her circulation and sensation checked and offers to use the bathroom or her need for fluids.

All was peaceful until 2:00 a.m. when she began to yell. I had anticipated that she would hopefully be ready to be discharged in the morning when it was light outside and my shift was ending. Her peaceful period sounded as if it had ended and was replaced by shrieking, "I want outta here, why have you chained me up, I didn't do anything."

Miss M.'s alcohol level was elevated way past the legal driving limit, not that she had arrived by a personal vehicle. Driving was often not an issue because many of our patients did not have access to a car. But their safety of walking had to be clearly known prior to releasing them. Her alcohol level was also not in the dangerously low zone, putting her in danger of having a withdrawal seizure. We were just waiting for

"Was my dress up when I came in?" she asked.

the urine and blood toxicology results, which would tell us what other substances she'd taken, resulting in her being our ONG (over night guest).

Although I explained this carefully, Miss M. wasn't interested. Her shouts got louder. For her safety, we put a leg cuff on her other ankle and then restrained her other arm. The normal response to being restrained on all four limbs is anger. Miss M. then became so angry that the gurney she was attached to shook from side to side. Just as I was beginning to believe that she would need chemical restraining, she peacefully fell back to sleep.

The woman was confusing, I thought. In between bouts of shouting about how she needed to leave and how dare we chain her up, Miss M. manifested another personality, this one cooperative and charming. "I'm so embarrassed that I'm here," she said, sounding for the entire world like a college sorority girl who'd just drunk her first beer. "Was my dress up when I came in?" she asked. "Oh, I feel so stupid."

Had something been slipped into her drink(s) that made this young woman so labile, I wondered. Or, had she been given some drug offered or given to her unknowingly? Miss M.'s violent outbursts alternated with her polite self. She continued to sleep, sing and shout. Because we still did not have all of her toxicology information back, she would remain with us for a while longer.

Around 2:30 a.m., always a busy time in ERs due to the bars closing. Miss M. quieted down. Miss M. seemed to have quieted down. So was the rest of the ER. I got a bite to eat, and around 3:30 a.m., I came into Miss M's room. I stroked her head, pulled her skirt down (again), and changed her into a hospital gown, when I realized then she had been *singing in the rain*, literally and figuratively. She was peaceful, so I decided to remove her right leg shackle. She smiled up at me and closed her eyes again, so I took off the right wrist shackle as well.

All was well, I thought. This young lady was well on her way to SIO and waking up in a good state.

She was checked every 15 minutes and then a little before 5 a.m., I went to check on her again. The room was empty.

The shackles so recently attached to Miss M.'s wrists and ankles were hooked onto the gurney. One dangled down from the top of the cart and one from the bottom, still swinging as if she had just vacated her gurney. On top of the gurney was Miss M.'s wadded up hospital gown. In the corner were her clothes.

Where was Miss M.? And what was she wearing?

I looked out in the hall. No one had seen her. I returned to her room. By now, five of us had gathered. Together, we looked wildly around outside of her room. Where could she have gone? The little room was maybe 8 by 10 feet; the only item in it a gurney. The walls were lined with acoustic white tiles, and the ceiling was made up of acoustic white tiles as well. We all looked around, and then, because there was no other direction left, we looked up.

Then we gasped.

One of the ceiling tiles had been moved over, and in the opening, we could see—it could only be—a woman's crotch. There was no doubt what it was. The only question was how "it" had gotten up there.

Miss M. was hefty, and this particular piece of her anatomy filled the entire opening left by the missing acoustic tile. We were all speechless, but the questions on all of our astonished faces were clear: How had she gotten up there? How could she *stay* up there, a hefty woman perched on thin metal slats? How on earth would we get her down?

The piece of anatomy was not moving. The body attached to it wasn't moving. Apparently, Miss M. had gotten herself up there and then fallen asleep again.

Someone giggled. And then someone else giggled. I giggled. Then all five of us were bending over, laughing till it hurt.

Sometimes—often—there is not a lot to laugh at in the ER. There are heartwarming moments, and often things to cry about, but rarely an event that will cause a roomful of ER staff to crack up. I didn't want to offend the woman's dignity, but it was hard to get a hold of ourselves as the little tiled room filled up with chuckles.

Then a different chuckle came from the ceiling. A deep, amused chuckle, clearly from the ceiling, or the person *in* the ceiling, but all we could see was a crotch. It was as if the crotch itself was laughing.

By now, all professionalism had flown out the window. The usual tension that accumulates on a night shift in the ER was releasing, big time, in our hilarity. A few of the staff members started making puns and jokes—the Voiceless Box, the Deep Throat from Down Under, and "Um, how are we going to get this Happy Hairball down from her perch?" were a few of the tamer comments. In the middle of this jovial exchange of one-upmanship, Miss M. began to sing.

"Love Shack ... everybody's movin', everybody's groovin' ..."

As we cracked up again, another loud voice could be heard from the next room. "What do ya' have to do to get a night's sleep in this booby hatch?" yelled a patient. It was, after all, almost 5:00 in the morning.

"I gotta pee!" came the voice from above. "And I'm HUNGRY!" After that statement came an explosion of gas, a warning of messier things to come.

We were stymied. "Who would have experience getting a stuck pussy out of a dangerously high place?" some jokester whispered, but then after that was out, the answer was clear. "Call the fire department!" Although we all laughed, we recognized the solution, because time was closing in on her ability not to pee. When one's shoe size was a nine or so on a one-inch strip of metal, and one was not wearing underwear, and one was still under the influence, no one could sustain the ability to "hold it just a few more minutes" as a female staff person encouraged her.

We concentrated on trying to devise a plan for if she fell—how we could soften the fall, for her and for us.

After the firefighters arrived, Miss M. let her feelings be known: she liked it up there! She had no desire to be helped down. No amount of reality checking could coax her to share less of herself through the ceiling. No one wanted to climb up there (although we tried to convince one young, cute paramedic to lighten his weight by removing his clothing and do his civic duty by climbing up and rescuing this maiden in distress).

For an hour, the only contact we had with Miss M. was with her *coochie* (her term, after she realized she was panty less). "I won't come down! I don't want to!" and so on. What finally brought Miss M. down was a bologna sandwich. After we offered it, we got to witness the improbable sight of Miss M. swinging herself down from the ceiling in a dainty, skilled manner.

At around that time, the patient's toxicology report came back. It revealed that there were no other substances in her body other than alcohol. Why she had acted in this bizarre manner for the past five hours, and how she'd been able to get herself up into the ceiling, remained mysteries.

Miss M. walked out of the ER as sweetly as she had entered, as if the night had never occurred, but for all of us on duty that night, she would remain the most unusual "patient presentation" we'd ever encountered—always good for a nostalgic laugh.

"If it's going to be funny in six months,
let it be funny now. A lot of us said this;
we thought we made it up."

CHAPTER 9

Drawer 14: A Cut Above the Everyday Bizarreness

Two nights before, we had a white man's genitals almost severed off, and that day we had a black set of genitals but no genital-less man.

WORDS OF AN ER DOC: *I've learned that my job is to believe everyone. If you come in to see me, you are there because you are in fear, pain and for right now, you need me to believe you. I want to believe you and I hope that you can trust me to take care of you. But I know that you may be lying to me, too. And that's OK, but wouldn't it be easier if you told me what you did put into your rectum, sir? But then I lie to you, too, mostly through omissions.*
—CORY SIEBEL, MD

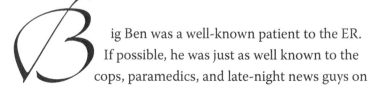

ig Ben was a well-known patient to the ER. If possible, he was just as well known to the cops, paramedics, and late-night news guys on

the street. As to why he was in the ER *this* time, his exploits all started from the time the Bio-Phone call came in to the ER from the paramedics with the short message "We've got Big Ben SOS" (SOS meaning "Same Old Shit"). All his visits followed a similar pattern. He would be brought into the ER somewhere between fighting someone or being totally passed out. He would sober up on a gurney in the hallway until he eventually discharged himself back to the streets. Often he reunited with a present or former best new drinking buddy while washing out his socks in the drinking fountain of the lobby.

The puzzle pieces of his life had never seemed to make complete sense to us in the ER. We felt we were pretty skilled at filling in the unspoken pasts of many of our patients' lives, especially the "regulars" (those seen once a month or more). Big Ben was an enigma. It was as if all of the border pieces of his life had been lost over time, and you knew that when the puzzle was finally put together, there would still be missing pieces. He never responded to our invitations to talk about his earlier life, so we just imagined what these pieces might look like. Truth mixed with make-believe. Sometimes it was our patients' truths or make-believe, and sometimes it was ours.

Big Ben sounded like he came from the East Coast, or at some time in his *little boy* past, there must have been a Boston or Rhode Island summer home. When he talked, his speech was garbled from too many alcohol withdrawal seizures when his teeth had chomped down on his tongue. His now permanently swollen tongue was like a purple-black fish in a small, old bucket.

He was six-feet-four-inches tall, lanky, blond, blue-eyed, and articulate after you learned to understand his delivery style. Every third word he uttered was "fuck." He could use the word as a noun, verb, preposition, adverb, double negative, or question. Someone even said that he could fart this word—and you'd know it when you heard it! He didn't own a car; he lived in enclaves: *under* places such as bridges, low-hanging street signs, bushes, turned-over shopping carts. In fact, he could even sleep standing up!

Big Ben sort of looked like Denver's version of the Marlboro Man with a limp. Jeans, cowboy hat and boots that we tried not to ever have to take off. He was always pissed off. You heard the anger, the vehemence, the dismissive way he spoke to sober people, which was completely opposite of the way in which he conversed with fellow alcoholics. Like many people addicted to one substance or another, he was scornful of folks that might have looked like him but were a *different* type of drunk or drug abuser—worse off or not as hard-core as he was.

Just when you thought you understood this man, he morphed into a foul-mouthed guy who had, as his most noteworthy characteristic, the dirtiest, most revolting pair of blue jeans we all had *ever* seen in the ER. The smell of detox (piss, vomit, sweat, and a yeasty bread smell that had gone sour) plus a street-gutter-grunge odor that clung to his skin and clothing was what most of us first encountered in Big Ben. The material of his jeans, we were sure, was *thicker* than any other blue jean material ever manufactured. Its thickness related to literally years of ground-in debris. If there really was a pair of jeans you "could stand up in the corner" (a phrase that never had meaning to me until I *met* Big Ben's jeans), these jeans were stiff with history.

To digress, Big Ben's jeans were like the blood I often drew from people with highly elevated cholesterol/fatty acids/ triglyceride levels. When their blood is allowed to sit for several minutes in the test tube, it turns an off-white color, slithers out of the collection tube, and it makes a "chink" or "chunk" sound when it comes into contact with the lab's metal counter. The material that clogs up some unfortunate people's arteries with high levels of cholesterol is comparable to the years of nonstop buildup of sludge of Big Ben's pants. We often spoke of culturing his pants because we had all been *exposed* to them and wondered what they might host that could be dangerous to us. We joked about how the next life-threatening bacteria or virus was probably in its formative stages right there, growing on Big Ben's pants.

He could never seem to pull up the zipper of his own jeans (why bother), but he could pick a lock like an expert.

We knew many of our severe alcoholics' pre-drunk, pre-downward spiral life stories. Learning about them helped us to learn about ourselves.

Over time, all ER staff members come to believe that most of us are just one to two paychecks away from what would be our own type of devastation. We take our own lives for granted, just as our patients must also have at some time. A medical crisis followed too quickly by a business failing followed by a love-life upheaval or a blow-up interaction that goes a little too far with a child, spouse, or boss all could create a pit, a failure from which many people are never able to recover.

I came in at 10:00 p.m. one evening, and Big Ben was already in the hallway where the SIO patients were flopped onto rickety old metal gurneys covered in ripped, nasty, black plastic. Most SIOers had one arm shackled to their gurneys (we affectionately called them "wrist bracelets"). Some had all four extremities *braceleted,* if they were on an EHH. The bars closed at 2:00 a.m., and after a big rush of activity from 2:00–4:00 a.m., it might be *quiet* until dawn, when all of the day traffic started. This is when we rechecked every patient, cleaned up, restocked, and hoped to "street" our patients.

Big Ben usually unconnected his own shackles. He could never seem to pull up the zipper of his own jeans (why bother), but he could pick a lock like an expert. I could smell him as he staggered past me to go to the hall bathroom even though his pee-soaked pants reflected that he had clearly failed to find a bathroom sometime earlier in the evening. He belched his way to clear an open space for him to sway past me as he headed for the "dick bowl." Usually he discharged himself from the ER and just wandered away.

He did, however, never leave before 4:30 a.m., when sandwiches were given out to the patients who had been the "nicest" to us (meaning those patients who had not given us a *hard time*). Everyone got a sandwich if we had enough. If we had fewer than four to six SIOers, everyone got lucky. The open hallways couldn't accommodate any more gurneys. Running the *gauntlet of sleeping drunks* was not unlike sidestepping unattractive furniture. They had "accidents," and cleaning up after someone relieving some part of his or her body publicly in the hallways could push even our limits.

The "triage" of resources is different in an inner-city, county ER than in a private ER. It is considered good business and the nice thing to do in a private ER to feed someone before he or she goes just as you would an overnight guest in your home. That night would have been a lucky night for Big Ben because we DID have enough sandwiches for everyone, even if he or she hadn't been *nice to us*.

When he opened the bathroom door, he mumbled something to me, but because my head was down near the floor emptying a gastric bag of liquid pre-shit material, I barely looked around because it didn't sound like fighting words. I decided to blow him off because his verbal shit (which I didn't need on top of the real shit I was dealing with) seemed sanguine. However, something in his voice made me turn around. Something wasn't quite *right* about this brief, grunting exchange. I took a quick look at him and noticed immediately that underneath the dirt on his exposed neck and face he was just a little too pale. His year-round dirt-tan couldn't hide that his color was just *off*.

"What's up, Big Ben?" I asked as I continued to size him up.

I was shocked at what the overly bright bulb in this tiny closet of a bathroom revealed. There was blood everywhere. I let the tired, old spring on the door close itself as I swung around and saw Big Ben start surreal, slow, then fast, sag to the floor. Big Ben became increasingly whiter, surpassing the fair skin tones I suspected he had always possessed, even though I had never seen him this color before. It was as if the years of dirt had just vanished. His color was draining away as the color of his infamous jeans quickly grew darker from the knees down. His low-slung jeans looked weighted down as the expanding line of crimson wetness grew. He slumped down as I pushed him backward against the wall to avoid a major bone-crunching face plant on the floor or onto me.

No other nurses, doctors, or cops going by noticed what had happened. Having someone plop down on the floor to "sit a spell" was not unusual. Having him keel over, all six feet four inches of him, though, was just about to happen and would definitely cause a big to-do in this overcrowded hallway. Big Ben had *done fell out* (DFO'd)—a term we all used that had originally come from black folks. This term was nonjudgmental. Women DFO'd from "pains down under," kids DFO'd, old people DFO'd. Folks DFO'd from bleeding, from "having hisself too much to drink," from the "sugar blood" being too high or too low, or from just being victims on their own or because of someone else's care-lessness, stupidity, or bad luck.

As Big Ben lay on the floor moaning surprisingly softly, I used one of my rare yells for HELP to compete to be heard in a hallway already filled with noise. Help came immediately. Two orderlies dragged his bloodied body up onto the nearest gurney, displacing the patient on it to a chair in which someone else was sitting, which we made him give up because he was "just a visitor."

Of course, the crimson pants and the bloodied handprints in a slithering pattern on the restroom walls set off my radar enough to yell "MAKE ROOM" as we pushed through to the main trauma room ASAP.

Big Ben did have enough energy to exude one big, loud groan directly in my face. As he exhaled a Thunderbird-reeking cloud of venom, I had the fleeting thought that approximately two percent of ethanol is metabolized by the lungs, and Big Ben's lungs seemed to be working just fine (and you thought that the horrific bad breath of drunks was just a bad hygiene thing!). "My dick!" he roared as he passed out. Where had Big Ben found a knife or scissors to whack off his wiener?

Let me take a minute to digress and explain detoxing to you from the perspective of a busy ER that operates with resources that do not resemble your home, where you can take one to three days to come down from a "good or bad drunk, bender, binge, or hard one"—where the desired effect is to get wasted, blitzed, juiced, lit, or fucked up. Depending on how he or she looks back over the unclear decision to drink as much as divinely possible, there are paybacks.

They know how it goes: sometimes they know exactly how much they've had, and sometimes no idea. We don't ask how much has been consumed because we assume they will lie (I'm sorry, but it's true), they are stupid (I'm sorry, but it's true), or they can't count because it serves no purpose to know how much (most likely).

All drunks have a favorite fluid, but every bad drunk will drink anything if withdrawal symptoms bear down on them. Did it matter? No, but we often had L-O-N-G conversations about brands of alcohol and their merits. For the life of me, I just couldn't remember then or now what Big Bens drink of choice was even though we must have talked about it over the five years I had known him.

As the team entered the trauma room, we all focused on getting him prepped for surgery. Minutes mattered. Every part of the human body has its own hierarchical position in terms of how much blood it receives. This has been determined through the evolution of our species based on supporting functions needed to survive. The brain, heart and lungs come first. The liver, kidneys and pancreas come next in importance. The blood supply to Big Ben's penis was of a high enough concern that wherever it specifically was on the hierarchy of organs, we knew he needed surgical intervention pronto, or he could bleed to death.

Big Ben had never before displayed any mutilation or overtly psychotic behavior. This was no time for hallway psychoanalysis, but I did believe I *knew* Big Ben, and this came out of the blue. There were two beds in the major trauma room. On one bed was lanky Big Ben, who had been "de-pantsed." We at first thought he had totally severed his penis because even seasoned staff gasped for a minute when there was blood dripping from both sides of a patient's gurney down the halls into the room. He hadn't completely cut it off, but reconnecting it would require hours of surgery with an uncertain outcome.

He was prepped in minutes for surgery. Life with a urine delivery system intact was the most the surgeons hoped for; they told him just prior to giving him a large dose of needed pain medication. No other pleasures or functions would probably be restored to him by our wonderful surgeons, but he would have his life.

After he was wheeled away, an unfamiliar, anxious vibe could be felt by those of us picking up from the previous eight minutes of chaos. No one had seen this coming. After he was gone, my eyes were riveted to his jeans, crumpled in a corner of the trauma room. I was sure we all were thinking; *now can we get rid of those jeans?*

Big Ben survived, and he left the Denver area soon after he was reunited with his urine delivery system. Maybe he had gone back to the place he called home with his crooked penis, we wondered? He had acquired legendary status. For years other hard-core alcoholics were compared with Big Ben in one way or another.

However, Big Ben's story, by coincidence, did not end here because it was forever tied to another event three days later.

The Case of the Missing Genitals

I was working in the trauma area of the ER when the sliding glass doors to the ambulance dock opened. Usually only ambulances with paramedics and cops brought patients through this door, but occasionally a screeching car zoomed in with a friend or family member rushing in exclaiming one of the following:

- "She's having a baby!"
- "He's been shanked (stabbed) or shot!"
- "I think he be dead, he ain't breathing!"
- "I don't know why he's not moving, and we have no idea why he's got all that blood on his head!"
- "I don't even know his name and (1) I just brought him in, or (2) I woke up and he was in my bed!"

On this day, two Hispanic boys, ages eight and ten, walked into the ER with a blue rag in their hands. They came up to me and tugged on my sleeve. I wondered why they weren't in school and figured that they had walked over from the park or the elementary school half a block away. They handed me the cloth and told me that they had found *this* in the park. I opened it up, and inside the dirty blue piece of old shirt material was a long (six inches or so), black penis and a pair of testicles. No blood, just a set of black genitals! They looked relieved that I was as surprised as they were, but ahh, the face of an experienced ER nurse is one of outward calm (I had had enough drama three nights before), and so I recovered immediately. They told me they had spotted this "package" lying in the leaves at the park and thought they should show someone.

Once again, in Trauma Room 1, there was a small "patient," another set of genitals—but this time completely cleaved from the rest of his respective body. I casually asked the boys if they had seen a body nearby, "like someone that might have been sleeping, drunk or dead in the park?" This question might sound strange if someone was asking it of *your* children, but in my mind I was formulating a possible crime scene. I led the two boys, who were after all playing hooky, over to a deputy sheriff stationed in our ER. The police, with maybe some help from my new pint-sized friends, might be able to help connect our *patient* to somebody, somewhere.

The "sophistication" with their *find* was something I had often noted in children who came into our ER. As crazy as this occurrence was (I had never been handed a set of cleanly severed off genitals in my life), they were as calm as could be. Life handed these kids experiences often macabre or bizarre to us. They witnessed events that had no references to my definition of *normal*, which they took in stride. This is how "street smarts" are acquired.

Two nights before, we had a white man's genitals almost severed off, and today we had a pair of whacked off black mans genitals.

Calls were made to the police. I figured that it was just a matter of an hour or so before some ER close by would be calling about their dismembered patient. In some ER, someone would come forward as a victim, dead or alive, to claim these parts. Till then, they were tagged (sort of) and sent down on a gurney to be placed in Drawer 14 of the morgue located in the basement of the hospital.

A year later they were still there, unclaimed. Their status eventually changed to "expired." They were packaged up in a pale blue surgical cloth (sort of similar to how they arrived) and sent to a long-term storage site downtown, at police headquarters, where other unclaimed body parts lifelessly waited to be reclaimed. We asked the cops over the years, "Hey, do you remember the day that Big Ben whacked off his wiener?" or, "Did anyone ever come forward to claim those other whacked off parts?" or, "So the infamous Drawer 14 *patient*, or at least his body, is still MIA?"

"Yeah," the cops would answer, "that was a strange couple of days."

Why have these two patient experiences been remembered as especially bizarre? When you consider yourself "experienced" or "seasoned," you can anticipate the risky patients who are risks to themselves or to us. Did I miss some slight behavioral change despite my self-perceived level of expertise? I had made a novice mistake. Dr. Peter Rosen states in his infamous "Rosen's Rules" his number-one rule: "Never think you can out-con a con or think like a prisoner, psych patient, or addicted person—YOU CAN'T."

I *knew* a lot about Big Ben when this incident occurred five years after joining the DG's ER, but I would never be able to anticipate, prevent, or know why someone chose to do a violent act all of the time. Maybe many times, but never enough of the time to ever lose my initial edge of fear, which *is* the behavior of an *experienced RN.*

These stories became intertwined because after the act of sexual self-mutilation had been perseverated upon, and no answers ever came forward, then maybe the mental picture of our "tiniest patient" in Drawer 14 provided a constant reminder (every time one of us had to go to the morgue) that we will never have *seen it all!*

~

Continuing to ask "why"
is the ultimate form of Control.

—Ron Hulnick, PhD

CHAPTER 10

The Clothing Boutique

No one comes into any ER with a change of clothing,
and many of our patients didn't have an extended circle
of relatives or friends who could bring fresh clothing
to the hospital.

The clothes that protect us serve as a uniform
that helps us assert our own identity, our aspirations ...
in our exterior are encoded the stories of our lives.
We all have a miniature living in a garment we've worn.
—EMILY SPIVAK

I t was Pam's idea, but as soon as she began describing it, all six of us standing around her started to smile, of course!

A "clothing boutique," Pam had said, and even as we smiled at the joke—boutique connoting something exclusive, whereas our patients' needs were so basic—we were already talking excitedly, our sentences overlapping. It would mean being able to put a fresh onesie on the sick infant who had puked all over, or to hand a clean blouse to the mother, or to give an unpolluted pair of pants to a person who'd been living on the street.

No one comes into any ER with a change of clothing, and many of our patients didn't have an extended circle of relatives or friends who could bring fresh clothing to the hospital. The need for adequate clothing was glaring, and we hurried to fill it. All of us began to search our closets for items that we didn't wear any longer. We asked our friends and neighbors for give-aways. We hunted out bargains in thrift shops. Soon, we had a decent collection of dresses, skirts, shirts, pants, and much-needed shoes of all sizes for men, women and children.

Underwear and socks were needed in all sizes. One day, undressing a 10-year-old girl, I recalled what my parents and my friends' parents would say when I was little: take a bath and put on clean underwear because who knows, you might be in a car accident. The understood message was that people in the hospital would see everything, and if your underpants were dirty or your socks full of holes, you'd be embarrassed. I believe that most of our patients also got this message, but *life got in the way*, and after a while they had to ignore or force themselves to forget this childhood parental edict.

The underpants on this 10 year old were ragged and skimpy. Much of the underwear we saw was torn, or dirty, or too big, or too small. The socks were in a class by themselves— frequently not matching and not new, based on their smell.

Many of our naked patients tended to have just left a wild party.

Often adults wore outer or underclothing that needed to be washed, but it is sad when a small child comes in wearing clothing that smells of sweat or oil, when their young sweat and oil glands are just developing and do not excrete much. These clothes have been on way too long—no changing into jammies at night.

The reasons our patients needed clothes varied as widely as the reasons they came to the ER. Trauma victims had their outer and underclothes cut off. Sick babies needed onesies and pajamas because their old ones were covered with, well, everything and anything that comes out of a sick baby. Many of our patients had blood all over their clothing from gunshot wounds or other penetrating weapons. What brought women into the ER frequently had to do with having or losing babies, and that often entailed a lot of bleeding. We needed lots of women's panties as well as pants to change into.

We also had a need to clothe those daring souls who entered the ER with a decided lack of clothing in the cold of winter. Men, women, and children would arrive without a coat, hat, gloves, socks, and shoes. We needed these items in all sizes. This was something I never expected but soon got used to. Folks sometimes arrived with simply nothing on at all. Patients arriving by ambulance were provided a sheet or sometimes a blanket to cover them if they were picked up from a scene, uncovered, but not all of them saw the need to keep covered with their *toga* sheets. Remembering to hold onto the sheet at the shoulders often went by the wayside.

Many of our naked patients tended to have just left a wild party. They couldn't begin to fathom where their underwear or bra had gone. As anyone who has ever been truly smashed knows, you sometimes feel an overpowering urge to remove an article of clothing because you're too hot, and then too cold, and then who cares, someone just dared you. The list of party decisions is endless. Removed with relief, the article of clothing often didn't cross the person's mind again until a trip to the ER inserted itself into the evening agenda.

The "how I got naked" stories abounded, in all seasons throughout the year. They made us laugh. The patients themselves made us laugh, weaving their way down the ER hallway, usually young and carefree and singing to beat the band. However, the situation lost its humor when the very same patients attempted to throw a punch at anyone who tried to escort them to a "nice, warm bed." As long as the swings didn't connect, we danced them down the hall and up onto a gurney, where the police, or physician, could then place them on a temporary, protective EHH.

The biggest reason we needed clothing was the most mundane: someone had peed or pooped in their pants. This did not apply only to little children. Bigger children had anxiety, and stomach issues. Adults fell into this category often if their alcohol level got in the .2 and higher levels. With that kind of brain haze, it's not easy to figure out when you're done in the lavatory either. Standing up too soon or forgetting to wipe a butt occurred far more frequently than one might imagine.

A one-time pee or poop might not be too bad, but the patients who did have this forgetfulness repeatedly ended up with something we called Bum Bad Booty. They smelled so bad that no amount of holding your breath and moving at lightning speed could offer an escape from it. All levels of staff that undressed patients just rolled up their sleeves and gave each other a *we're up to our necks in alligators so we just have to wade our way through the swamps look* (this saying usually ends with draining the swamp, but this we knew would take too long when all we wanted was to get out of the room ASAP).

It was not just their clothes that smelled so strong. "P and P" that had made its way down into shoes and socks—or up the other way, under the waistband, creeping into all the skin's crevices, set up a home that after a few days begins to reek of decaying flesh. If skin is left unwashed for too long, and an opening into the skin occurs, a simple infection can then progress to becoming gangrenous. This type of infectious process has an easily identifiable red-brown skin and a distinctive odor. Rarely does anyone have to ask twice, "What is that uniquely foul smell?" You never forget it.

When new clothing was offered, you would think patients would willingly strip off the old stuff and accept the new, but that wasn't always the case. Just like little kids, some of the patients stripped with little or no encouragement, but even though we showed the gloriously clean shirts or pants with which we were going to replace their soiled ones, some fought us. We didn't want to battle over clothing, so we gave them their soiled clothing back in a bag.

What made the struggle interesting was that sometimes, in the course of removing old clothing, we did come upon buried treasure. The most common item was a half-smoked cigarette, and the second most common was a joint. These were hidden in imaginative places on the body, the fat fold of a tummy being the location of choice. Other places to hide a rolled-up cigarette or smoked-down joint were the groin, the butt, and inside female genitalia. If we absolutely didn't need to check those orifices, we chose not to. *Go ahead, keep your joint.*

Sometimes X-rays would reveal these little surprises. We often didn't know of illegal drugs or a spare bullet until viewing the X-ray where the person complained of pain. Then we would see a wad of something tucked back there. We were fine with it staying there until the patients were discharged.

In various other locations we found plastic-wrapped packets of cocaine; money (bills and coins both); small pieces of paper with phone numbers or locker combinations; betting slips; lottery tickets; and not infrequently, odd pieces of jewelry—an earring, ring or necklace. Why the individual wouldn't be wearing said jewelry, I wondered? Then after a while, I got used to the idea that the jewelry was stolen.

We also found sentimental objects, for which I had a soft spot. This could be anything from a religious item to a small baby spoon. Not infrequently, I found photographs—in a locket, or pocket. I always tried to make sure these items were placed in a patient belongings bag with his or her name and hospital record number affixed to it so the treasures would stay safe.

Jewelry, as well as clothes, had to be taken off if we believed it would get in the way of the physical exam or an IV, or it was in an area that would be X-rayed, sutured, or put in a cast. We explained to patients that we bagged and tagged everything we found on them. Cash was logged separately and taken to the hospital safe.

A surprisingly large number of individuals never dreamed they would later become patients the night they happened to be wearing their "favorite" parka, jeans, or roommate's sweater. High anxiety would especially occur if the item they had on still had connected sales tags from the "five-finger discount" tucked discreetly out of sight. It was not unusual for patients even in a lot of pain to yell strict instructions: "Do not cut off that shirt" or, "Those are my good-luck jeans, for Christ's sake!" How lucky indeed—you are now in the ER!

Depending on the suspected level of trauma, we tried to remove jeans without cutting them. That was often harder, and more painful, than they or we wanted to endure. Often the clothes were already splayed open from the paramedics doing what they thought was necessary during the ambulance ride. No paramedic or nurse wanted to be the one who missed the gunshot wound

(GSW) or stab wound (SW), because he or she obeyed the patients' instructions not to cut off their favorite jeans.

All victims of sexual assault, men and women, needed underwear and something to wear over their underclothes. It was really for these patients that we started the clothing boutique. Giving one's clothing to these patients was a seemingly small act. "There but for the grace of God go I" was often what I silently prayed to myself—and that they would never be in this vulnerable situation again. Clothing, a vestige of autonomy, dignity, and non-vulnerability, is a value held by many. We saved any new underwear we had been given for these women. It was one more reason to love the clothing boutique.

Within two weeks of our announcing the idea, the boutique was brimming with inventory. Relatives, friends, and neighbors had contributed generously. We had designer labels along with recently dry-cleaned and still-bagged items that almost seemed new. Even the well-worn articles of clothing had to be presentable. Our policy was to accept only clean items in decent shape. Our bottom line was, "If you wouldn't consider wearing it, then we won't accept it."

> To human beings, the meaning of clothing is deeper than the functional purpose of cover and protection from environmental elements.

The boutique was a lively place. Clothes were constantly taken out for various patient *events*. Sometimes recipients would travel back to the ER weeks later, wanting to return the items they'd used. Sometimes a recipient would bring in other articles of clothing, a contribution, in the spirit of giving back.

Occasionally, former patients of ours or people who had heard about it from another woman in a shelter came by because they had no appropriate clothing for a function they needed to attend.

"I'm going for a job interview, and I need a suit," a young man might say, having been discharged from a halfway house. "I need to attend my mother's funeral, and I have nothing nice to wear. Can I borrow something?" was especially poignant.

One of the sweetest requests came from a young pregnant girl. She'd come into the ER for a rash and confided that she was on her way to the courthouse to get married. A few of us nurses spent a happy half hour helping this bride-to-be and later her betrothed, who was meeting her at the ER, choose their wedding outfits. "Le" clothing boutique resulted in their choosing a pretty summer dress for her and a "real nice coat and tie" and tennis shoes for him. We waved them off with wishes for a happy life together. And $32 collected and put into his coat pocket.

It was definitely not a fun job to get the assignment of "straightening out the boutique," which is why we took turns at this task. Even though we began with clean clothes, sometimes an individual would don an item, decide it wasn't "right" in some way, and then put it back, along with some little critters recently living in that individual's hair or armpits. It's not easy to get rid of lice, scabies, or nits when you don't have a hot washer and dryer to kill them, but that's what we had to do.

Sometimes we had to delouse ourselves, however hard we tried not to get infected. I always took a shower as soon as I got home, so I was surprised one day to realize that the itching in my armpits was actually some uninvited guests. I used the same over-the-counter (OTC) medicine we gave to our patients. This was another experience that elevated my empathy level. It is so easy to blow off some seemingly minor-sounding complaint until you, too, have suffered the same. I had all the modern conveniences: a washing machine and dryer in my home, a good shower, and money to buy more medicine and new sheets. Our patients didn't have these resources. It was doubly hard for them to obtain these simple items, so they often became reinfected.

The boutique revealed in a subtle way a change in how staff members became more empathetic with regard to how people were dressed. There had never been outright callousness about someone's clothing, but now any jocular comments were met with a "look" that nonverbally communicated that the speaker was not funny. A child age four or older who entered our department with a parent, wearing pajamas in the middle of the day, always tugged at my heart. A child this age knows he or she is not dressed appropriately and does feel embarrassed. Maneuvering around to say something like, "We have a few too many shirts and pants that I think might fit your son perfectly. Would you like to take a look and see if you and he like something? It would help us out." It worked for me, and I hope for them also.

One nurse in particular, Georgia, could make any patient feel like he or she was a gift to us. She worked in several homeless shelters in town, and when she was on duty, the number of people who went to the boutique increased significantly. It was not just the clothing with which they walked away. Georgia, more often than I think we realized, would sneak a $10 or $20 bill in a pocket, wink, and say, "I think you got an especially nice pair of pants there, Mister."

Georgia gave this money from her own pocket whenever she felt a patient could use an "unexpected gift from a stranger." She liked to think of them using the $20 bill for a "real meal in a real restaurant." Georgia always said she thought the most important thing was people knowing someone out there cared. People more often felt that if you gave homeless people money, they would spend it on drugs or alcohol. "Maybe some did—but some didn't," she'd say as she was walking away, and you caught a quick wink from her.

The rules of the boutique were that you took only one of an item and only what you needed, but sometimes we bent those rules. A 12-year-old boy once selected a red velvet shirt with a satiny collar that someone had brought in. I happened to be there at the time, and it intrigued me to see a young boy appreciate this item. I thought as he picked it out of a box with "Medium Shirts" written on it that it looked like part of a stripper's costume. His mother had other ideas. "Pick somethin' else," she said. "That is a *whore's* shirt." The boy's older sister joined in, "That's a dumb choice. What you pickin' up that thing for?" she laughed.

The boy refused to put the colorful shirt down, but then another nurse came in, saw the boy holding the red velvet item and guided him over to a "guy" shirt in his size. The boy looked distraught. I went over and, winking at him so he'd know I was up to something, handed him the "guy" shirt at the same time I took the red shirt from his hands. His eyes followed my hands as I first held the red shirt behind my back, then stuffed it in a plastic bag, then handed it to him. The boy grinned and stuffed the bag beneath his coat. To his mother, who had seen the whole thing, I said, "If it's okay with you, it's okay with me that he has it—a gift."

I always wondered what the boy did with that shiny, soft shirt. Did he use the fabric for something? Did he dress up in it? Did it just make him happy to have it in a plastic bag? I hoped it brought him happiness. If only because he got something that he wanted.

To human beings, the meaning of clothing is deeper than the functional purpose of cover and protection from environmental elements. The subtle impact of suggesting that a woman having a pelvic exam keep her socks on decreases anxiety by alleviating one more area of potential worry of inadequate hygiene. Clothing is also a symbol of our culture and our place in that culture. It represents choice and the expression of one's self. When we first started the clothing boutique, I saw a girl choose a cute burgundy T-shirt that happened to be one I'd contributed from my own closet. I'd bought this top on sale, and I was happy to see this young girl pick it out to wear. When she walked by, I told her, "That looks really good on you."

"Oh, this shirt?" she said. "I got it out of the rag bag in the back. I can't imagine anyone paying money for this. Nurses have got to have THE worst taste in clothes."

I had to laugh. I really had liked that shirt. Hmm, I hoped this wasn't true, but I had to inwardly smile, thinking that I also might have said this at 18 or 19 to cover having to wear a stranger's discards. I understood this response. I realized how my pre-conceived idea of someone rejoicing over wearing something of mine "couldn't be that bad," but it probably was.

I tried to set aside any items from dying people's bedsides and/or effects, imagining that their next of kin would be delighted to get them. This might be, I reflected, but just as likely, all of the attention I gave in this type of clinical presentation might not be important at all. If there was a possibility that something like an article of clothing might ease the pain of not being present when their loved one had died, it was worth it to me to continue to believe that this area of perceived control, by me, made a difference.

Finding, in some small way, a connection to lift up the dignity of which many patients in our environment came in with a deficit, was not difficult. The challenge was to provide what might be needed with respect, sensitivity and kindness. The clothing boutique was not about making us feel better for giving things to people in need; rather it was an opportunity to gain humility by better understanding what compassion looked and felt like.

Before you know what kindness is
you must lose things, feel the future
dissolve in a moment ... all this must go.
Before you know kindness
as the deepest thing inside,
you must know sorrow as the other
deepest thing. Then it is only kindness
that makes any sense any longer.

—NAOMI SHIHAB NYE, poet, songwriter and novelist

CHAPTER 11

Intimate Strangers: Dying Is a BIG DEAL

There is nothing like the deep connection
and reverence we feel when someone
has passed on in fulfillment of their destiny,
even if we have just spent the past hour
or two fighting this outcome.

*Spirit threads are words that once inflicted,
often cause pain, which then creates a
'heart-wound' which then becomes a guiding scar
and guiding star—transforming a perceived wound
that often heals beautifully.*
—DAVID JAMES DUNCAN, novelist, *The River Why*

I have learned a lot about dying: passing, moving on to the little sleep, the Big Sleep, flat lining, the forever city, the point of no return, Freedom! going home in a box, feet first, all the way, coming home, pushing up daisies, the body farm, the bone yard, the last roundup, cashing out, checking out, taking the endless sleep, the last pit stop on the highway of life, a place of peace, going home to be with Jesus.

There are so many euphemisms, so much jargon and slang, for the process of dying and the state of death. ER staff members are aware of why they default to words and phrases irreverent to macabre. The choice of descriptive words can have the power, even if just temporarily, to convert a crisis situation into a manageable event. Death in an ER differs greatly from death in a hospice or home setting, when there is a little bit of time to prepare for what appears to be an impending death.

As surprising as this comment might be, in fifty years of being a nurse, I have never worked on a "floor," a medical surgical unit with medical and/or surgical subspecialty patients, although this is the public's image of a nurse and what she or he does. I am a "critical care nurse," having worked only in ICUs and ERs when I worked in hospitals.

In an ER, the fast-paced rhythm often demands that there be an efficient, coded style of communication to get everyone on the same page. Alerting each other with a quick term has the power to shift gears so that we can be in synch to perform the tasks we each have been educated to do. We are here to fight against your dying, your death. Quickly responding with the life-saving skills and behaviors that become automatic to us can be set into motion by the group dynamics of those around us. Words or phrases can become similar to rituals for some staff members.

Most of us are quiet, and although our responses might be different, I know that each shift, each team always seems to find a way to listen, respond, and act unified in their efforts toward the common goal of helping to keep a patient alive. A verbal utterance can prepare some team members to quickly get into the aggressive mindset they need to perform their tasks. As shocking as it might be, "Let's cut this meat wagon off the road before we find ourselves rolling in the rotten carcasses headed for the glue factory" quickly allows some to distance themselves from the procedures they are about to perform on your body, to fight death from taking you in *its* clutches.

My role does not include amputating a person's leg or drilling holes through someone's skull to alleviate permanent damage to a person's injured brain or delivering a dead baby from a 50-mile-an-hour, blunt-force auto accident that spared the mother. This helps me not to judge what I hear.

We cannot physically distance ourselves from the intimate pain your battle to survive will impose on us both. There is no real humor experienced by anyone in the ER when someone's life is tragically or painfully unfolding. Code talk can provide a sense of defense, some armor to help protect us during the upcoming battle that you and we are trying to gang up on.

Dramatic language can motivate some staff when all of the physical resources have been used and the thought creeps in that we might be losing this battle. Then, when every medication and piece of equipment has been tried, sometimes over and over again, the use of these powerful sounding, bravado words slows down our impending sense of failure. With each round of drugs or interventions applied to keep us winning this desperate foot-race, our fear is that your reserves will give out before we can wisk you over the finish line.

> Too many times to count, we have all seen patients that *should be dead* from the description of what happened to them, and they make it.

It might seem odd that some staff members use language to push back against being cynical, hard, or non-caring. Humorous words can serve to especially distance some staff members from patients deemed as deserving to some degree their impending deaths. If their negligence, substance abuse, or intention of violence lands them in the ER, or their carelessness resulted in

injury or the death of someone "innocent," I have seen humor
sometimes used to stop a staff person from crossing the line into
unacceptable anger, the real emotion, and that may be harder
to personally manage.

When the ambulance delivers a patient to the ER, and the
doors are flung open, and the gurney is snapped up, we are all
immediately visually assessing you for pain, fear, and your level
of awareness. When we see fear in your eyes and that you are
able to scream or cry, we know that this expression can mean
many things. Your cries evoke in us the deep desire to first
decrease any pain or fear that we assess you are experiencing.

Patients are brought in with their clothes and belongings
still clinging to them as if to say, *I have a story; I am not history
yet; I have not passed on.* People in auto accidents or traumatic
falls or with gunshot and stab wounds are often picked up on
the streets as "scoop and runs." They are delivered to us:

- We look at their trauma, and we look at their response
  to the story we were told as to what happened to them.
- We look into their eyes.
- We believe that they can hear us even if their eyes are
  shut, and they are critically unstable.

Too many times to count, we have all seen patients that
should be dead from the description of what happened to them,
and they make it. When the opposite happens, this reinforces
to me the mystery of life and that we have never really been in
control of who lives and dies.

We don't always know the stories behind the events that
bring some of our patients into the ER. This is often best because
it supports our pledge to preserve your life to the best of our
abilities no matter the reasons for you being here with us. Not
knowing prevents filling our heads with junk that we just don't

need to be thinking. It is hard not to be judgmental when you hear a horrific story. Sometimes ignorance helps to prefill the space I might be filling with angry thoughts. Even if my thoughts are unsubstantiated, revengeful thoughts, they fill my need to find a person or a situation to blame in an effort to advocate for my patient. My thoughts don't have to make sense. They only serve to temporarily answer *why and who* could do this to another person?

After experiencing a major traumatic event, many of our patients are still conscious and alert. For the most part they are desperate for just a little more time. They are living, hoping, and fighting, and then suddenly they realize they are dying. Their response to their own realization that death seems imminent is verbalized in "NO—STOP—WAIT—PLEASE—NO." There is sadness, anger, unbearable grief—a vast range of human emotions that spills out like the blood from their wounds.

As death becomes more likely, there is often a desperate desire to connect with someone, anyone. The connection is frequently by touch and eye contact alone. If they are young and victims of trauma such as auto accidents, I attempt to hold onto some piece of them (a hand or a foot) and to speak or murmur some words while holding as much uninterrupted eye contact as I can. Not separating, even with what may be the most minimal of connectiveness, is huge when the noise, pain, and focus of all the people around you may be saving your life, but you feel alone and desperate.

Most of us see the actions of a caregiver as parental, what we would want someone to do if this were our child or our loved one of any age, is primal, not just compassionate.

Children sometimes ask, "Am I gonna die?" just as adults do. When I am responsible for providing the answer to this pleading or panic-stricken cry, for a split second I am unsure of what or how much to say. Then I do *know* what to say. I hear the words spoken, and I listen from my heart. Depending on their age, my response might range from "I don't know" to explaining every action and consequence, but the constant message is, "You won't be alone. I'll be here with you. Hold onto my hand."

I don't know if this is the "right" or "correct" path to take. I do know that I listen to what my patients are saying. Many patients will tell you exactly what they need or what they want you to say to a loved one. We know that you are someone's wife, mother, father, husband, child, or friend. You and I are now intimate strangers, and because your path has intersected with mine, we have a sacred bond. Our connection feels transcendent, I am honored by being present in your life.

None of us would come back and do this painful work if we didn't empathize with our patients. Over time most of us do get "good" at responding to dying and death, outside and inside. We are able to fight for someone's life, win or lose, and then move on to the next patient.

"Why did this happen to this little child? What meaning does this particular death have in the cosmos of this family? This is so tragic. Life is so unfair." These are all thoughts we will come to terms with later. Occasionally, developing the skills to face death daily can involve becoming harder or more insensitive to protect oneself, but this is rarer than you might think. And over time, attempting to be tough and unfeeling takes its toll by creating pain in the lives of the people that love us.

We don't always win the battle.

After a patient has been pronounced dead, there is rarely any time to reflect on what just happened. The room is a mess. It takes us all; the housekeeping staff, nurses and doctors to restore the room for the next patient. As gruesome as cleaning up all bloody equipment, trash and organic remnants of your losing battle to evade death, this time gives me the opportunity to stay in the room, to quietly feel sad, frustrated and consider what brought you into the ER and who was now taking up the struggle of suffering because of your death. I gather your belongings, which often will provide a link to your loved ones of your final time here, such as clothing you were wearing when you transitioned from living and breathing to no longer speaking, crying, hoping, or struggling.

If you die, we all *know* that you are still *here* with us in the room, afterward. Not just as a covered-up body but as a presence we feel as you continue on in your journey where science, skills, and those of us still physically present in this room are not needed and have no expertise.

We know death is universal and irreversible, and there are no treatments or cures for death. After death has occurred, there are no more medical or nursing actions we can take to fight for you, to stop, to win over the path you are now on.

It's difficult to speak of dying in impersonal terms even when relating a story. Yes, we all do become "good" at performing tasks that end in the resuscitation room resembling a battlefield. Bodies that have been gruesomely opened all reveal stories of how those holes were inflicted.

For us to stop pushing your death away can also evoke thoughts that we did not do enough to "save you." This is not true, but these thoughts have been compared with survivor guilt in other situations where one person for whatever reason dies, and the other person doesn't.

Accidents, injuries, and fate are no strangers to us either. Most of us believe and hope that someone would fight for our lives if we were in your circumstances. Battling for the victory of life that successfully overpowers death might not be what all patients want, and when it isn't, we listen to the plea for us to stop. We don't always stop because we know that fear and pain can cause you to plead with us to stop. We don't stop when we believe that we can see beyond the corner of your being overwhelmed ... and that our actions will result in your individual life continuing on past this difficult time for you.

There is nothing like the excitement and joy experienced by everyone when a woman precipitously gives birth to her baby as soon as she comes into the ER. Similarly, there is nothing like the deep connection and reverence we feel when patients have passed on in fulfillment of their destiny, even if we have just spent the past hour or two fighting this outcome.

When you experience birth and death with someone, the impact of the mystery of these events is such that you know it doesn't matter if you knew *a lot* about the person or not. In the most hopeless times of our lives, we often must depend on strangers to be competent and kind. Intimate strangers are the separation between life and death for you and possibly will be for us also.

> *"Anytime you take strangers agony*
> *into your own body, you are changed by it,*
> *refined into a vessel better able to give*
> *and to receive love."*
> —MARY KARR, English Professor and author, *The Liar's Club*

CHAPTER 12

Jackson and Guillermo: Dying up Front

I hoped, like I always did when I couldn't hold
my sadness inside, that this involuntary response
from me did not make someone's loved one
lose hope.

*The Storyteller's Creed. I believe that
imagination is stronger than knowledge,
that myth is more potent than history,
that dreams are more powerful than facts,
that hope always triumphs over experience,
that laughter is the only cure for grief,
and I believe that love is stronger than death.*
—ROBERT FULGHUM, author

As I was walking into the ER with Jim, an orderly, and two nurse friends, Marion and Meredith, we all were chattier than usual. Our gait and our pace were exuberant, and we laughed about how a particularly arrogant resident had been chastised by Dr. Peter

Rosen, our distinguished ER director. We had to temporarily stop our gossiping because of the loud sirens of not just one, but two 911 ambulances close behind us as if to say, "Hurry up, you guys. It's a hot Saturday night, and we've already started bringing them in!"

So much for being early, I thought to myself.

"Am I gonna die? Am I gonna die?" I could hear as soon as I stepped from the locker room into the hallway leading to the front triage area. No report again, I thought as I remembered that I hadn't put my lunch in the refrigerator, and I hoped the broken headlamp in Room 23 had been fixed and there would be enough laceration packs in Room 3, unlike last night. Whew, five minutes into this place, and I was already prioritizing my own multitasking thoughts!

I heard overhead, "We need you STAT, Julie, in Trauma Room 1."

Doctor Bill, a third-year ER resident, was probing the abdomen of a lanky young man with not just two fingers, but almost his entire hand (a gunshot wound or stabbing I wasn't sure because the amount of blood all over him and the floor almost meant that at this time it didn't matter).

Because the paramedics had already placed two large bore IVs into the patient's arm, and an intern was trying to examine the rest of his naked body for more injuries, especially holes, I grabbed a Foley catheter to put into his penis as he was just about to be sent STAT to the OR. With all of the pain this terrified man was experiencing, it didn't seem as if this procedure could elevate the noise level or his thrashing about any more, but it did as soon as I grabbed his penis! His hands, strapped down with soft but strong Kerlix restraints to keep him from touching his wounded abdomen, came undone. He violently grabbed my hands.

"Stop him, Julie. I've got to see how deep this wound is! He's not talking, so I'm finding out the old-fashioned way; I'm digging around for bullet fragments until I can get him over to X-Ray," Bill yelled at me.

"Hang in there, Kid, I know it hurts. What the hell happened to you anyway? It would help a lot if you told us," snapped a surgeon who came in to eyeball the patient into whom he would be making more cuts in the next 15 minutes in the OR in an attempt to save this young man's life.

Patient: "Oh Jesus, NO, it hurts so bad, give me something. Am I gonna die?"

Me: "You have just been stabbed in the gut, and we are all going to do everything possible so that you will live."

Patient: "Is my wife here? I gotta see her. Please stop—STOP!"

Me: "There is a lot going on, and you are seriously injured, but if she is here, we'll go get her. If she is not here, what would you like me to tell her?"

Patient: "Tell her I love her, tell her to tell the kids, tell my momma that I love her!"

Me: "I will."

Patient: "Will you pray for me? I can't believe this is happening. NO, no, stop, stop!"

Me: "I will tell them, Jackson," I said as I saw a piece of paper with his name on it.

I was frantically looking around to ask the orderly to retie Jackson's hands so that I could get the Foley catheter in. A second orderly, Marcus, quickly tied Jackson's hands down to the gurney that would transport him to the OR. I somehow got the catheter in with all of the movement going on as each team member quickly finished his or her tasks. The urine coming out of his bladder into the 1,000 cc collection bag looked like pure blood, not yellow urine. This was bad. The stabbing, which looked like it had created a huge hole, had. The wound when he came in looked big; after his 10 minutes in the ER, it looked like he had a lot of damage internally.

"Jackson, your wife is not here, and you are going to the OR. I will tell her that you love her," I said as I moved my eyes inches from eyes that confirmed his pain, fear, and frantic desire to escape from being tied down on this gurney going to the OR.

"No! Wait, I need her so bad now! Wait a minute—till I can see her, touch her," he wailed, but now in a voice with a new element of realization that eclipsed the pain of his stab wound—the sound of primal panic. A wail, a moan, anger that can't go anywhere and dies somewhere in the exhalation of air, his eyes straining for any different path or place to be but here. Beginning to realize that his words of defiance were not affecting all of the craziness swirling around him, did not *really* seem to include him evoked the desperate look of a dying man, but a man who was going to be much alive up to the minute of his death.

"We can't wait, Jackson—give her a kiss on this paper, and I will see to it that she gets it," I thought up moments before his gurney was pushed to the elevator to take him to the second floor OR. The door made a heavy click, click sound as it zoomed to the OR on the second floor, and I held what might be a last piece of connection Jackson has made here on earth.

"Stop—don't forget to give it to her," I heard as the elevator door closed.

An hour later, we heard that Jackson had not made it.

I had the bloody scrap of paper, the wrapping around an unused but still bloody four-by-four-inch cotton dressing I grabbed off the counter for Jackson to clench onto as he kissed the paper in agony. I placed it in his patient belongings bag, knowing the social worker on duty, thankfully, would protect this paper and share it word for word with Jackson's wife when she arrived. Because it was still only 11:30 at night, and Jackson's wife might not have been informed to come to the hospital when the social worker or I was here, I hastily scribbled a note to accompany the patient belongings bag: "I took care of Jackson before he left for the OR. He wanted you, his children, and his momma to know that he loved you all. This paper is a kiss that he wanted to give to you." —Julie

I wanted to say more, do more, but I knew the bloody clothes we cut off Jackson as soon as he arrived, in addition to his shoes and T-shirt, had to be picked up and placed in the patient belongings bag. All of these remnants of Jackson's final living moments would be given to his wife. Not surprisingly, these items often meant the world to loved ones.

The room looked like a battle zone. There was congealed, darkening blood, Jackson's blood, all over the floor, mixed in with paper wrappings and stainless steel medical items we separated out to desterilize and those items that could cut us. The desterilized instruments would be used on someone else's life, with a different outcome than Jackson's, I hoped.

Next door in Trauma Room 2, I saw five staff members working on a patient whose body I could see only as an adult, black male. This time there was no blood, but there was the same intensity of intermittent, loud talking among staff members stating either their orders for someone to carry out or the results of an action they just completed. To someone passing by this room it might have appeared from the staff members' facial expressions, or a curt-sounding voice, or the look of total focus on the technicalities of performing a particular task that no one seemed to be responding to the patient's feelings of hopelessness.

I considered going into the room to help for a minute or two, or to be with the patient, but just then I saw at the head of the bed my friend Meredith.

I saw Meredith putting in an IV and drawing a blood sample from the line while talking directly to the patient. Although I could not hear her, I knew from having worked with her that she was telling the patient what she was doing and what the results were of his EKG. Everyone else was looking at the changing EKG rhythm, recognizing that this patient's electrical conductivity was dangerously progressing to a complete heart block (going from bad to much worse, from the standpoint of this man's heart). Meredith knew this, but she was looking at the patient as she was also pulling the pacemaker out of the core cart. Core carts are in all of the major resuscitation rooms, and they hold the most emergent medications and equipment for when your heart or breathing has stopped.

I didn't linger because Meredith appeared to have it all under control. Meredith is kind, and she is highly competent. Life-saving actions related to medications; EKG rhythms; intubation; airway management; and charting the blood, vital signs, replacement of fluids, and procedures, along with the patient's responses to every one of these interventions, would get done. Staying connected to the patient's need to know what is going on, if he or she has pain, or if he or she wants to tell us something is a role valued by everyone on the team providing care. Nurses often are designated for the role of staying in tune with the patients' understanding of events—are they fearful, do they have questions, or was the term SOB used, which to us means short of breath but might be distressing to the patients hearing this said about them!

My attention was diverted by a non-911 ambulance bringing in a woman in a wheelchair holding a pale little boy wrapped in a thin blanket that smelled like vomit and diarrhea. "Mijo, Mijo," she exclaimed as she held him to her and rocked him as if to transfer energy from her anxious body to his lifeless-appearing body, alarming to her and to me as I passed by and saw him looking too far away in a permanent outward, non-blinking manner. His eyes appeared to have fallen to the side of his body being intermittently hugged to his mother's almost equally foul-smelling, stained blouse. One quick look at her, and it was obvious she had been caring for the *cachorro* ("little puppy," as she lovingly called him) for several long days and nights.

"This four-year-old little boy has had vomiting and diarrhea for the past three days and is SSO," the paramedic told me as the child moaned and spit up some vile-smelling, green-brown material.

Not knowing he was Spanish-speaking only, I looked to the mother and asked her if he had a fever. She did not reply, and the paramedic stated, "No one speaks English."

I pointed to a pediatric bed as I guided the paramedic pushing the wheelchair to the closest of three beds in the room. I asked Jim, the orderly walking by, if Marcus could come and translate for me until I could find a translator in the department. Oh, please let there be a translator on duty tonight, I thought to myself even though I didn't recall seeing a name on the assignment board when I had come in just one hour earlier. Working with a translator would make getting a detailed history of this little boy's illness easier, but until one arrived, *cachorro*, my four-year-old little patient, needed care immediately.

Guillermo's mother and I unwrapped him from his blanket while we could all barely conceal "holding-your-breath" facial expressions at the pungent and dreadful smell. More worrisome was his diaper, overflowing with liquid, green-brown fecal material —and this looked and smelled like what I saw coming from

Guillermo's mouth. He needed washing, but I needed his diaper removed so that I could take his vital signs and examine him. "Cuanto malo? How long bad (sick)?" I asked in grammatically poor Spanish.

Mrs. Gomez acted out vomiting by moving her hands from her stomach to her mouth over and over and said, "One week vomiting and four days' diarrhea," as she pointed to his bottom. Guillermo quietly moaned, "No, no ...."

I took his vital signs. His temperature was 104.7 rectally. This came as no surprise because he looked parched: "You are so hot and dry, Little Man, that you can't even make sweat and pee," I said softly to him. I thought Mama knew what I was thinking as she saw me feel his skin, and with all of the poop in his diaper, no one would know if there was pee mixed in with the poop. We looked into each other's eyes, and we both knew that her son was very sick.

His pulse was 176 (normal for his age is 80–110), and I was glad we had a pulse-oxygen device to measure this as it was racing up and down, making counting this fast of a pulse almost impossible. Mama and Papa were watching my lips, and their heads bobbed slightly as I counted out loud, 76, 77, 78 in the first 30 seconds.

Guillermo's respirations were 40 (normal are 16–24), and they were shallow, short little gasps that literally looked like a fish out of water making little sucky sounds. "I can't hear his blood pressure," I said to the orderly. "Let's take him to Trauma Room 1." I was unable to obtain a blood pressure in the room because there was talking, and I knew that if it was in the range I felt more than heard, then 40 over 30 is supercritical.

I scooped him up and headed for the second bed in the resuscitation room as I called out to a passing physician that I needed a doc immediately. There was a patient from an auto accident in the other bed. Under ideal circumstances, we wouldn't have used the second bed in this room, but this is why we had this bed, *just in case. Guillermo was the just in case.*

Grabbing IV tubing and a bag of normal saline, I quickly placed a tourniquet around his nonresistant arm. I can do this, I said to myself. I've done this hundreds of times on equally—no, even sicker kids. However, getting IVs into severely dehydrated patients is tough no matter their age. I've done this a thousand times—please, God, let me have this stick, I said silently, just as I could hear the wordless hope from the other people now in the room wishing or praying the same.

To my surprise I got blood back from the stick, but I could not insert the catheter. The physician also tried and was unable to get the IV in Guillermo's arm. His vital signs looked worse. His heart rate was continuing to go up even higher. His blood pressure was continuing to go down, and he was now not gazing or blinking. This child is going to die, I said to myself, knowing we were all beginning to think this. I grabbed an acetaminophen rectal suppository and put it quickly in his hot rectum. It melted immediately, but I knew he needed a heart that would pump this medicine around for it to even have a chance at lowering his dangerously high temperature.

An interosseous device was placed in his leg—one we use when the patient is in *extremis*, when we need IV access to provide fluids and medications. Placing this device involved forcefully jamming a needle into the child's upper thigh bone. Another physician entered the room to place an IV in the child's neck. This took several minutes and was successful, but the child now no longer had a blood pressure or pulse.

I had known Guillermo, his mama, and his papa for seventeen minutes.

"Come on, come on, Guillermo," Jim the orderly said as I showed the boy's mama how to cradle his head because we were all around every other inch of his body, which might have only had minutes of earthly life energy in them. She did not move after she anchored herself to her son's body. Papa was rubbing his son's foot, but he kept on having to move to make room for someone who pushed him away. There was only so much room around his little child's body.

We all listened to the cardiac monitor as cardiopulmonary resuscitation began, which his parents and the staff could hear that his formally fast rate was now starting to slow down. All of the staff members' faces looked focused and determined, unlike those of his parents, who frantically looked only from my face to Doctor Bill's, beginning to realize that the life-saving fluid was not going to deliver the magic that we hoped our actions seemed to promise when we started.

"Mijo ... Mijo ...," his mama intoned.

Doctor Bill began barking out orders for medications as an anesthesiology resident who appeared from nowhere placed a breathing tube into Guillermo's tight, inwardly puckered mouth. An intern whose name I didn't know began chest compressions, and the realization was obvious in Mama and Papa's eyes that their son was *in a place* he wasn't in a minute ago. I believed that both parents felt God in the room with them and that heaven was now opening itself up for their son.

All of our bodies and faces were inches away from each other's. We didn't need a translator anymore because words weren't needed. We were all connected to one another, and there was a feeling of reverence as we continued to give more fluids, more meds, more oxygen, and continued compressions, all believing that in just a second he would turn the corner, and the monitor would show his heart beating, and his limp body would move ever so slightly.

I felt my own eyes tear up, and Guillermo's mother saw this. She had been crying softly and I hoped, like I always did when I couldn't hold my sadness inside, that this involuntary response from me did not make someone's loved one lose hope. It could, I knew, but not usually. For me, it always means that I am moved by the life-and-death struggle with which I am involved. How often does this happen—maybe once a month? I don't fight it any longer.

When another staff member is experiencing an intense emotion, we all understand why this happens and have confidence that each of us will pull ourselves right back into full, head-on, high-functioning mode. In an ER setting, we as nurses and doctors are fulfilling our obligation to you to maintain, restore, and improve what we can, for your physical body to remain alive.

Desperate glances and kisses by his parents continued, in addition to our CPR efforts, for another 50 minutes. The room smelled sweaty, and tension appeared on everyone's face—but no one wanted to stop helping Guillermo's heart to pump the medicines and fluids that still might have meant he had made it up and over the mountain of staying alive. Life might have been slipping slowly away from little *cachorro,* but the conviction of *in just a minute more he will turn the corner and be okay* was evident on everyone's face.

Doctor Bill asked the person doing the chest compressions of CPR to stop for 10 seconds. The line on the EKG machine went flat, and the room was immediately silent because there was no beeping sound coming from the monitor without the chest compressions being done by the medical student who had relieved the first intern 20 minutes earlier.

"We have done all that we can," Doctor Bill stated in a voice different from the commanding voice with which he had been giving orders for the past hour.

"I am sorry, Mr. and Mrs. Gomez. I wish we could have done more for your son," he said directly to them as he touched both of their shoulders and then softly stroked Guillermo's leg.

It was evident that Guillermo's parents knew their son had died. The medical student, the other physician that entered the room half an hour earlier, and the orderlies all touched Guillermo's parents as they murmured words to them that I hear but would also be saying when, in a few minutes, I was alone with them and their son.

I turned down the glaring, incandescent light overhead as I stayed in the room with his parents, and we gently washed his little body. A soft baby blanket donated to our clothing boutique was brought in to cover him. All of the tubes, IVs, and the interosseous device had to remain in place because Guillermo's death was an "unexpected death of a patient not known to be sick or under the care of a physician" and would be considered a coroner's case, a case in which an autopsy would be performed. I wished that we could take away all of the evidence of the battle to fight off death, the battle we had lost, but we couldn't.

The Gomez family would never have enough time with Guillermo, neither that evening nor ever. I knew they were numb with pain, and they did not want to separate from their son's body; their need to protect their son from some ongoing pain or trauma did not stop when the monitor said that his heart had stopped. Every minute would be forever seared in their minds, and it would just never be enough time. They crouched down to the floor as his body, now covered with a sheet, was wheeled from the room. This final good-bye is so painful that none of us ever gets "used to it."

*There are few human expressions more genuine
than a cry of grief. We don't have to wonder
what that person is experiencing.
It is the soul revealing itself,
right now I am broken.
Grief is not deadness, it is feral energy.*

—Francis Weller, psychotherapist

CHAPTER 13

Sex and the City

We women bonded silently with each other
when women patients were overpowered
and abused by men.

*There are many ways to victimize people.
One way is to convince them that they are victims.*
—KAREN HWANG, author, *The Humanist*

ack then, all of us nurses were women except
for Dudley and Fred. These two were the type
of men that made us all welcome men in our
female midst. They were two of the most sensitive men, who
reinforced to many of us that nursing was not something that
could be entirely taught. It was something "in your DNA,"
meaning that you had the "caring gene." Although all of us in
the ER—paramedics, residents, physicians, and nurses—bonded
through our intense experiences, we women bonded silently
with each other when women patients were overpowered and
abused by men. There really was no male equivalent for the men
in our fields. Sexual assault does happen to men, but women are
the primary victims of this crime.

We nurses had seen each other through falling in and out of love, bad breakups, marriages, miscarriages and divorces. All of us knew how to be calm in the face of chaos. We had come to experience upsetting accidents as the reasons we were here and our life's work. However, when a woman was brought into the ER because she'd been sexually assaulted, it never felt quite like "business as usual." The deep, primal fear, the powerlessness of women subjected to this specific violation—all of us felt this in our shared vulnerability. We also felt anticipatory anxiety because we knew that after she entered the hospital, the woman was going to feel like she was a victim all over again when answering questions that invaded her privacy. We knew something these women did not.

If the victim first called the police, she was instructed not to change any of her clothing or wash off her body, the two things all victims are desperate to do.

After a woman enters the hospital claiming to have been raped (and it *is* rape whenever she says no), it is only an alleged rape until evidence is collected, and this sets the stage for the judicial process to follow. Gathering evidence for a crime scene sounds simple unless your body is the crime scene. Proving allegations of rape, the forceful entry of one person into another, involves obtaining evidence that must provide the roadmap of every activity of the perpetrator. Swabs are taken of any orifice penetrated, pubic hairs are plucked from the victim, and then the pubic area is combed to pick up any other hair that might have come from the assailant. Pictures are then taken of any area of the body that appeared injured—this is one of the most embarrassing and difficult parts of the exam to have to endure.

No matter how many exams I participated in, "No" means No. Forcible, unwanted intercourse is difficult to sometimes judge. The "truth" is in the data gathering process. It makes me cringe for the patient and sympathize with her as she described every facial expression, word uttered, and minutest detail of the assault that took place. Perpetrators words to their victims often reveals the truth of the description of rape as a crime of violence rather than of sexual desire.

The police officer who is often the first one to see the victim begins by questioning for agonizingly thorough details of what happened from the first moment of contact with the perpetrator. The beginning of the assault is when some women lose track of the events that follow.

Victims of trauma often become overwhelmed quickly by the shock, fear, and feeling of powerlessness at being grabbed, thrown to the ground, punched, or threatened by a weapon. This fear creates a powerful fight-or-flight response that short circuits memory. Recollection of the details needed to piece together a rape experience tends to be more accurate if obtained as soon after the event as possible.

A woman survives the attack only to undergo the physical exam that follows, invasive by its very nature, and, depending on the assault, sometimes painful. A woman comes bravely forward seeking safety in the supposed haven of a hospital and in minutes, questions and fingers are prying into areas that are numb or are screaming out *no*.

One August evening stands out to this day. What was the statistical likelihood that I would be the nurse who supported the data collection and emotional support of five different women who came in after being sexually assaulted? Each had a different, horrifying story to tell.

The night shift began at 10:00 p.m. Soon after I arrived at work, a pretty Hispanic girl entered the clinic with her mother, who still wore an apron and had a flushed look to her cheeks and perspiration on her forehead as if she had just popped something into the oven. Both were in tears.

"I snuck out of my house to meet this boy," the preteen girl said, in between sobs. "I saw him at the mall. He seemed nice, and he had a car."

The car that the girl had admired—and foolishly got into that night—took her to a park just a mile away from her house, where the boy who had seemed so nice threatened her with his fists clenched right at her nose and eyes, hissing, "Don't you dare scream. Remember that you came with me." Sexually inexperienced, she was looking forward to her first kiss.

"As soon as I closed my eyes, he hit me in the face and tore off my pants," said the young girl, who then threw herself into her mother's arms and sobbed. Sharing just these details resulted in complete shock.

As much as I hated to break up their embrace, we had to do our exam as quickly as possible. We covered every part of her that we didn't need to examine, to maintain her modesty. Murmuring softly, the girl's mother held one of her hands, and I held the other while I got her positioned on the exam table. I kept eye contact with this traumatized girl as I did what I had to do to support the thankfully female physician on duty who would be conducting the exam. However, nothing could diminish the girl's anguish right now. The sight of her innocence utterly destroyed stayed in my mind, knowing that this would be a memory that would never get completely erased even if she was able to get the most supportive love and therapy.

Several hours later, just 15 minutes apart, two women in their early 20's entered the ER. Both had endured a sexual assault in different parts of downtown Denver. They didn't know each other, but they had made exactly the same mistake: each had linked up with a man she hardly knew, hoping to get to know him better. Each had subsequently said "no" when the man wanted to have sex.

Each had been raped and would arrive in the ER with different police officers, unaware of the other. Each felt entirely alone as she stood there with blankets around her, which the police often gave victims even if it was a warm night like that night—it offered protection of another kind. The details didn't matter as much during the transfer of the patient by the police to us in the ER. This is often a quick report. "She called us, and we picked her up at a friend's house," but we know that standing there in a busy open lobby when she is often in pain, hurting from the sexual and physical assault, she just wants privacy. The look of shock is often followed by humiliation as she hears her story being repeated to a hospital staff member.

"I can never trust a man again, ever," the first woman said. She was a slightly plump pretty woman working as a per diem secretary. "How can I go back to work? How can I face my parents?" she wailed. Although she then became silent, I could imagine that the "what if's" were piling up in her own mind.

We went into the cubical, not even a room with a door that closed. If we had any one-patient rooms with a door, all of us would have designated that room as being for SA (sexual assault) patients. The ER was old and rooms with doors would not be available until several years later.

The police officer waited outside, and I asked the young woman if she knew that I would need to take all of her clothing because I could see that her skirt and blouse were torn and dirty. As much as she no longer wanted these remembrances of her attack touching her skin, it was difficult to take these items off. I had a warm blanket (thank goodness the blanket warmer had been stocked even though it was summer and often the meager eight blankets it held were used for trauma victims). Clothing is always taken into custody as evidence. It is the first barrier of separation between the victim and the assailant and provides valuable forensic evidence that tilts the story in one direction or another in a she-said, he-said allegation.

When I asked for her clothing, albeit one of the least embarrassing parts of the exam, was when this woman seemed to wake up. I wasn't sure if she was mildly intoxicated. The police officer told us he had picked her up in a booth at Denny's.

Seeing the shame in her eyes, I tried to comfort the young woman while assessing that she had been slugged in the eye, had her clothing ripped off of her, and she barely was able to raise her left arm without help. As I helped her undress, I said, "This wasn't your fault."

I knew it wasn't her fault, but often a sexual assault will leave scars of self-doubt that affect a woman's life for a long time. I have heard the "what if's" extend beyond what if I had been more seriously hurt or died to include the inevitable, "Why didn't I fight back harder; why didn't I scream?"

The other woman entering with her was intoxicated, and although I removed her clothing and gave it to the police, she was unable to provide any information other than, "I'll kill that SOB for fucking with me. I didn't even know the guy, I just met him," or variations of a barroom event of which details would not even have the possibility of coming forward for several more hours.

She was covered, and a physician on duty came back to attempt a history and physical exam but could only report that there were no obvious signs of trauma at this time. The police report was that she had hailed an officer off of the street, stating that she had been raped. The official complaint would have to wait a little longer before she was able to give consent that she wanted an exam to collect evidence. She would not be leaving, and the "evidence" would be safe because she was unable to wash herself.

It was around 2:00 a.m. when we nurses were just recovering from the coincidence that I had somehow been the nurse available for all three sexual assaults, when another woman—we found out soon she was 58—entered the ER. She came in alone. This mother of five and grandmother of eight—her name was Kate— had lived in the same urban neighborhood for 17 years, on a street that had a drive-through alley behind it. That alley contained the dumpsters for residents to deposit their trash.

That night, Kate went to put her trash out in the alley, about which she had long had trepidation. "I always knew something bad would happen to someone out there, one of these days," she said, "because drunks and drug addicts were starting to hang out." What Kate couldn't have imagined was that a gang of boys her son's age would have set upon her, ripped her skirt off, and raped her.

Kate had not had intercourse for 20 years. The boys left her raw and bleeding. "I'm an old woman," she said, bewildered. "What would they want with me?" I had no answer for her, just a comforting hug and a clean skirt from the clothing boutique. She did not want the underwear. Her daughter and a son came in to take her home just as we finished the exam. "Don't call my daughter till I'm ready to go home; I don't want them to be frightened and upset," she stated. "I'm still their mother."

It was the fifth woman's story that really rocked me.

As we each tended to our patients just before the sun was about to peek down the streets, a 28-year-old, newly unemployed woman about to return to Minnesota, Sarah, was still in a bar on Larimer Street in downtown Denver. It was 4:00 a.m., and the bars were supposed to have been closed for two hours. The new bartender did as expected. He closed the doors of his establishment at 2:00 a.m., but he told the few patrons left—Sarah, another woman, and four men—that they could "stay awhile."

Sarah had been drinking, but she was "still in control," she said later. A short time after the other woman left, Sarah got up to leave, but the four men blocked her way. They pushed her into a back room and told her she wasn't going anywhere. In minutes, Sarah recalled, they had stripped all her clothes off. Then one by one, they raped her.

As she told what happened next, Sarah's body and voice shook violently. After they raped her, the men laughed drunkenly, forcing a wadded up, plain, brown paper bag over Sarah's head. They told her to bark like a dog, and when she wouldn't, they kicked her. Oral and anal rape followed. "You know you love it," the men yelled at Sarah the entire time.

It went on for hours. When the men were done, they threw Sarah—naked, bleeding, and incoherent—outside. A stranger saw her and called the police. Paramedics brought her into the ER wrapped in a blanket. Sarah did not want any male to touch her, not the police or the paramedics or a doctor.

Then Sarah had to endure the sexual assault exam.

She kept her bruised, swollen eyes shut as we worked. I told her in as soft a voice as possible what we were doing each minute. "You can tell us to stop at any point," I said, but she never did. Even though she moaned throughout, Sarah cooperated with our evidence-gathering procedure.

When asked if the men had ejaculated—a standard question—Sarah had no idea. The physician and I looked at each other over

Sarah's head. There were tears in his eyes, I saw, and I knew there were tears in mine, but there was more to come. The pain Sarah still suffered was so intense and the level of humiliation so high that she could not report the other vile things the men had said and done to her. It was not until we physically examined her that we discovered teeth marks on Sarah's thighs and strangulation marks on her neck. Two fingers on her left hand were fractured, as was her right wrist.

"I'm never going back home now," she whispered to me as she lay covered in warm blankets, waiting for the orthopedic surgeon to take her to surgery. "No, please stop asking me if I want someone to be called. I don't. I have to do this alone." I sat by her while she dozed, waiting for a surgery room to become available. My thoughts and feelings I willed to be stopped. This place I had gone to before when there was nothing more to do. I just needed to be present.

We have come a long way in terms of how victims of sexual assault are treated. It used to be that women were blamed—for being a tease or for the clothes they wore or the choices they made. A lot of misogyny lay under those beliefs.

Now, we consider it a rape if the woman has said "no," and the man continues. Now, most ERs that see a lot of sexual assaults have sexual assault counselors who came into existence in the 1980s. These are often laypeople who have taken courses in the ramifications of and procedures surrounding rape. They are there to emotionally support women in the critical period immediately after they have been assaulted and to help them through the exam when crucial evidence must be collected to catch the rapists. Many of them are rape survivors.

Prior to the SA counselor's presence, nurses were the only staff who could serve this purpose, and often, in the middle of comforting a rape victim, we had to leave the room to attend to another emergency.

Sexual assaults are heinous because the effects from them cannot be undone or easily forgotten. Sarah, I knew, would be followed by social workers when she came out of surgery, but this is often not the time when the victim is able to process the trauma. Sarah might be able to overcome this night of terror, whether choosing to live in Colorado or Minnesota, but I would never know this or the outcome of her or any of these women's rapists being found, convicted, or punished.

That summer night, when five different women who had been assaulted were brought in—when they sat there in their cubicles, their own clothes in tatters, bagged as evidence—I did what we all did back then when the effects of these types of patients on us, their caregivers, was not yet known as PTSD. I distanced myself from my fear of this type of thing happening to me by believing that these events happened to "other people," not me. This was wishful thinking, stupid really, but it was all the recourse I had available.

We did feel their pain, so much so that it was hard to even talk about it among ourselves.

That night, I remember thinking how glad I was that we'd established our clothing boutique. We had a stock of new underwear donated, and for cases such as these we saved these brand-new items. It seemed like a small thing in the context of what these women had gone through. These women had been stripped of their dignity as well as their clothing. Giving them fresh clothing along with the empathy in our eyes and compassion in our hearts was a way of saying, "You don't deserve what happened to you; you deserve respect."

We did feel their pain, so much so that it was hard to even talk about it among ourselves. I didn't want to burden my friends with the details of that night. They had experienced similar episodes of women in pain. It wasn't that I was tough, it was that maybe they had had a tougher, more painful, or sadder night than I had experienced. I told myself that my night could always have "been worse."

If rape did ever happen to me, I thought as I drove home that morning counting the minutes till I would reach my own warm, safe bed, at least I knew what would happen, and I wouldn't be like my patients who had no idea of what was going to happen when they came in to be seen and cared for.

Some say there is a constellation of behaviors.
I know there is a unique footprint
we are each born with and grow into ...
I know what it's like to be without a Self
and what it feels like when that Self returns.

—Carol Denker, author, *Autumn Romances*

CHAPTER 14

A Tale of Healthcare in America

"Arima mundi – the soul of the world
is trying to speak. It's telling us that its
capacity to mend itself is at risk."
—Francis Well, author, *Navigating Our Losses*

t was sometime in July, on a shift that was almost too calm for eleven PM. Would it rev up to be one of those "full moon" shifts that emergency room staff don't really believe influences "crazies to come out?" This night didn't feel like it had the potential.

With its bullet proof glass doors, the main ambulance entrance to the ER looked like a department store loading zone with high concrete walls and big black bumpers attached to the back-up wall. An occasional screeching car would drive into this area with a woman delivering a baby, or a victim of trauma that someone has raced to the hospital to *unload*, but did not want to stick around for. *But not tonight*, I thought as I looked at my refection in the doors.

Until around midnight.

Any private vehicles to this area results in our deputy sheriffs coming out to "meet" you. They appear quickly. Depending on what you are dropping off, deputies can be a *good* thing or a *not so good* thing. If it was your purpose is to "Drop and GO," or "Load and Leave," then these eagle-eyed men might alter your departure plans. If you indeed did want immediate help, then these men, with big muscled arms could look like angels from heaven being there to envelope you to safety.

Under layers of dirt and his deeply tanned shoe-leather skin, it was impossible to tell if he was forty, fifty or sixty years old.

A slow moving, old, wood paneled Chevrolet station wagon, with filthy, dust covered windows that looked like it had been driven from somewhere in the outback in Australia, creeped into our Ambulance Only area. After watching the driver attempt three different times to back into the dock, two sheriffs hopped down the three foot embankment and walked over to the driver's side window. With one hand on their holsters the deputies were ready for anything.

Two deputies flanked the car, coming up from behind, one at each front door. Each opened a front door at the same time. All we heard was, "Jesus God, what is that terrible smell," as they backed away as soon as the doors had been opened.

The deputy on the driver's side did not need to ask the driver to step outside of his car. He just fell out.

Under layers of dirt and his deeply tanned shoe-leather skin, it was impossible to tell if he was forty, fifty or sixty years old, even under the bright lights that automatically turned on as they detected movement.

One of my favorite deputies, Ben, asked the old man. "What brings ya here?"

In a voice that did not seem to match his appearance he replied, "Well, I don't rightly know what you can do here for my old man. He's an *old as dirt geezer*, who's in the back here. Till we all decide, I sure would love a drink of water if you can spare me some."

"Where are ya from?" Ben asked the man with the young voice. Chuck, another favorite deputy of mine, who appeared to possibly never have cracked a smile in his entire life—but who was uproarishly funny, went back to the station wagon, took a deep breath, and then peered back inside to take a look at the "old geezer."

"We've been driving from Phoenix" the *old-young* son stated, in between taking a final long gulp of water from the plastic disposable urinal that we often used as water containers since we were always out of paper cups. The man that we only knew as someone's son motioned to have the container refilled with more water.

Once he had downed close to a second liter of water, he related to us that the drive had taken two days, non-stop to come to "y'all."

The drive from Phoenix to Denver, even in a car that looked like it was on its last legs, is usually no longer than a sixteen hour drive. Non-stop driving for forty-eight hours made us all wonder as to why this trip had moved at the pace of the Bataan Death March of 1942. Going through the desert, day and night and day and night in the heat of summer, with a passenger that we still could not see, but assumed had not been much help with the driving, opened up all of our curiosity.

But first, if our driver had just drunk close to one thousand cc's of tap water, then presumably his passenger, his father, was also thirsty. This journey was beginning to suggest that indeed, a survival feat from the desert was about to unfold.

Two orderlies, Marcus and Jim, trotted by with a gurney headed to the pavement to assist 'Moses' from the back end of the station wagon. After wrestling with the jammed latch that might not have opened with ease for the last ten years or more, we waited for what, we weren't sure.

A bunch of trash, an old duffle bag and one empty pop can rolled out and clinked to the ground as the orderlies reached in to retrieve Moses from his years in the desert. Just then Marcus and Jim began pulling a make shift aluminum device that looked like a piece of bent, discarded, ski patrol equipment used to take people down from a mountain top, we heard this deep, rumbling, gurgling, gasping for air noise come from *father*. He was bundled up in several old, woolen blankets, even though the inside of the car was roasting hot. "The air conditioner gave out the first day," the *son* mumbled. The old Army/Navy blankets were left in the cavern of the car and replaced by our yellowed blankets that often looked old and dirty, but just now looked very white and clean.

Carefully Marcus and Jim extracted a man with no clothes on except for a deeply stained tee shirt with "Texaco—you can depend on us to get you there safely." ironically splashed across the front of it.

The smell of urine, old food, and caked on moldy-sweat is what everyone was struck by as *father* was wheeled by, tugging the blanket on the gurney all around him such that even his eyes weren't visible. *Son* sat down on the three foot embankment and said "I hate the old man, I gotta go," as he languidly headed for the street corner traffic light. Someone said "Whoa there ..." but I didn't hear the rest of the exchange as I headed back into the ER.

I was the assigned Charge Nurse on for the shift, and had only come out to the ambulance dock area when I saw the red brake lights of this car flash on and off so many times. Once we got our patient that still did not have a name, into the department, I assumed my non nose-breathing style of talking.

Son must have been "encouraged" to stay by the deputies, because he reappeared, still holding his plastic urinal bottle of water. Sweat that is the result of extreme physical activity often has a "clean" smell to it as opposed to sweat that is coming from someone that has been in an extremely tense and prolonged state of panic or fear. *Father's* sweat that had started in Arizona was probably a lot older than the two day old trip. This man's sweat, to this day, remains the most hormonally charged, fight-or-flight level of pungency that even his equally competitive urine smell came in a distant second.

We knew that *son* probably wanted food and rest, but we needed to hear how and why this odyssey had been undertaken.

"We came to your hospital because my shit-for-a-father was discharged from a nursing home in Arizona. I ain't seen him in a long time but he tracked me down," he cryptically stated. *Son* paused to take a bite of a bologna sandwich that someone found and had given him to eat.

"What's the matter with him?" Ken, an ER doc asked as he followed the patient into the room. We didn't know how sick *father* was but gurgling an unintelligible answer when asked "What's up" will result in you being super quick.

After devouring his sandwich *son* became more talkative. "He can't breathe. He's fifty and too young for Medicare and until this last month, not sick enough for Medicaid. He was discharged from a hospital to a nursing home, but they turned him out like a dog even though he can't barely breathe right," *son* told us in one long, exhausted out-of-breath sentence.

We temporarily were calling him, "Mr. Down and Out." We used this phrase when we didn't know a patient's name. It carried a degree of respect indicating that someone had experienced a lot of bad karma or luck, but they were hanging on fighting against unfavorable odds. It was not condescending. "*Bad luck and bad juju,*" we often all said, could happen to anyone, but it often felt like it was not fairly distributed. It implied strong resilience, strong DNA and some luck along the way.

"When the old man found me, I knew I had to git him some help even though he's a rotten son-of-a-bitch," *son* told us. "I met some guy who was practically giving away" an old 1965 woody station wagon and "my old man and I scraped together the money to git him the hell out of that sorry ass state. "

The next time I popped into the room, both men had names. There was no social worker on to navigate an ability to pay and because the patient had no proof of residency in Colorado or anywhere, this is when I *loved* my hospital. Someone had given this father and son good advice. *Go find a hospital that takes people with no money*, so they did what they had to do. Desperate times require desperate solutions.

Richard and son Daryl had decided to go to Colorado when he was kicked out of not just one nursing home, but three, when the nursing homes had met their state's legal obligations to provide care. They did not want to have to provide care "forever" for someone with no recourses to pay anything toward his own care, and was a non-Arizona resident to boot! A guy at the gas station a few blocks from the last nursing home suggested going to Colorado where it was "easier" to get care. Daryl took off looking for some necessities for their journey to Colorado, a state that neither of them had ever been to before.

He found a suction machine from a third tier, resale-market shop in Arizona that sold used hospital equipment. Most of the stuff was long out of date, or wrecked up, but if a buyer wanted to take a chance, then this was the store of last chance. Daryl then went by a trash container outside of a sports store and found a bent frame of what must have been a dog sled (of no value in Arizona) for " the old man to sleep on." And off they headed for I-25 North to Colorado.

What they did not in their innocence expect or foresee would all occur.

Daryl began to relate their *father-son* story to Marcus and Kimberly, a nurse that left shortly after summer ended, stating "this place is too much." Somewhat surprisingly, Daryl helped us in removing his dad's oily tee shirt. Kimberly removed the mayonnaise jar wedged between his excoriated legs. Urine had spilled out of the Mayo jar onto his skin, many miles back. Empting the jar came secondarily to his need to be suctioned for lung secretions that he just didn't have the energy to cough up and out. And probably hadn't since before he left Phoenix.

The little suction machine (which was really meant for a small animal veterinarian clinic) would conk out if it was used for more than ten seconds, within a ten minute time frame. Richard needed suctioning before they had gone five miles from the gas station on their way out of that "state that ain't got one ounce of decency."

The car had been packed with what Daryl supposed he would need for a sixteen hour drive to Denver. Four plastic bottles of water, some sandwiches, chips and two candy bars.

The suction machine was going to be powered by the car lighter and a connector that Daryl bought at a flea market. It came with one single use suction catheter.

Thirty minutes out of Phoenix, which was really not "out of" Phoenix since it was rush hour, and traffic was moving at a pace that made "me feel antsy right at the get-go," Daryl pulled over to the side of the road to suction his father after he had a particularly deep, fulminating cough that produced so much mucus that he started to sputter and not be able to talk. The "tube got clogged up, I didn't know what to do so I just blew out all of the yellow-green shit," he said with a sigh.

For the first three hours his dad required suctioning once an hour. To clean the catheter, Daryl told us that he used some of the water from his small cache of water to rinse it out, "... and blow through the top end to help dislodge the stuck-on stuff."

I came in out of Richard's room whenever I walked by because I was drawn to this family unit. As bizarre as they appeared to be, they still functioned as families *should.* Kimberly had started an IV to give him much needed fluids, suctioning him and medicating him for his high temperature of 103. I felt a sense of dread reflecting on the cross infection that must have occurred between Daryl and his father over the last forty hours of being in a small space with his father's coughing, no hand washing and reusing the same single use catheter over and over again.

All families are unique in how they live together or apart throughout their lifetimes.

As soon as *dad* was settled in our Observation Unit waiting for a bed upstairs, where he would be suctioned, given fluids, food and skin care for the red, raw skin (which explained why he didn't have anything on from the waist down), Kimberly had Daryl sign in to be seen. Daryl's temperature was even higher than his father's. Daryl vital signs reflected, if possible, that he was sicker, with pneumonia than *dad* was.

This acrimonious family unit needed medical care and financial assistance. And they needed someone, someplace to be kind to them.

When we all got off of work in the morning, we headed over to Denny's to eat breakfast and fill each other in on the details of Richard and Daryl's desert odyssey.

Father and a son had driven across the desert in a thirty year old car, stopping every twenty minutes for the last forty-eight hours to get to a hospital, in another state just because … just because they had to. Like his dad or not, this son had done the right thing. He could have walked away many times from his father.

All families are unique in how they live together or apart throughout their lifetimes, but Richard and Daryl were especially unique. Choosing to stick together and not abandon each other is a decision that I admire when someone in the family does what they may not want to do, but does it anyway.

Just as I had learned years before that no one grows up planning on being addicted, penniless, homeless and alone, this family expanded my understanding of how the struggle to survive is infinite. Over the years I witnessed many families figure out how to be there for each other. And if someone's biological family became lost or destroyed in some way, not everyone was able to create new families that provided strength and protection from the toughness of life, but many did.

The year was 1987, and now thirty years later we, an immensely rich nation, are still struggling to provide healthcare to every person in America. Patients and their families still reveal that they have been forced to move from state to state seeking care that they couldn't find where they came from. Healthcare is regionalized in America; what is offered in some states does not exist in another. Many patients do not know the "rules," the guidelines, the criteria for how to get the care they need. Being turned away creates a migration of people picking up and taking off to seek resources in the form of jobs or healthcare very similar to the 1940's movie, *The Grapes of Wrath*. Healthcare is not yet *right* for many in America.

We are living all too often in the Great Forgetting.
We've forgotten that we need each other.

—Daniel Quinn, cultural critic

PART III

THE DISCOVERY

"The attraction and disenchanted factors."

CHAPTER 15

Camelot: Why Nurses Stay and Why They Leave Camelot

These ingredients create an ideal environment for a human being to become his or her best self and to look for new frontiers that beg to be explored ... and don't feel restrictive when you feel you are just getting started!

Don't let it be forgot
That once there was a spot
For one brief shining moment
That was known as Camelot!
—CAMELOT, THE MUSICAL, 1967

*C*amelot, a musical by Alan Jay Lerner and Frederick Loewe, is based on the King Arthur legend. The modern-day interpretation of this place symbolizes the epitome of civilization, chivalry, romanticism, order, and progress. *Camelot, located nowhere, can be anywhere.*

As I climbed up each rung in my career ladder, I experienced new challenges, each of which taught me something, caused me to enlarge my skills and broadened the breadth and depth of what a registered nurse could accomplish. All of my stories up to now—from my choice to attend an old-fashioned, Catholic, all-girls nursing school to my 30 years of practice—were filled with excitement and pride.

Looking back on the first thirty years of my career, the phrase "Camelot Nursing" comes to mind.

The notion of Camelot has been used not just in the Lerner and Lowe musical, but in cultural references and speech, to represent a place or time where certain elements come together to create a sort of perfection. The usual meaning of Camelot is the epitome of civilization—romanticism, chivalry, order and progress. But my nursing colleagues and I used Camelot to denote a special place where we could be the best nurses ever.

"Camelot, located nowhere, can be anywhere." It was used by film critics in the 1960s to describe this fantasy place that *could be real.*

When and where did the term Camelot Nursing originate?

The summer of 1993 was a time of high gang violence in Denver, with more murders taking place than in any other time in the city's history. As the summer wound down, one night at DG we all ended up staying for hours after our shift should have ended. We had to restock and clean up before the cleaning staff could do their thing. That late night Pam alluded to our work situation as Camelot. She did it in jest—but we all understood her meaning. That night, that summer—all levels of staff had worked in synch, all of us giving care so fluidly, working together in such unison, that we all knew we were inhabiting an elevated level of professional care.

Those summer months would not look ideal to an outsider, but the moniker stuck. For us, "Camelot" came to represent a work situation that captured the real reason we'd all wanted to become nurses, and the reason we stayed in nursing when it didn't.

"Camelot Nursing"—when everything seems like perfection: not because the experiences are all positive; not because the tasks are easy; or not because the patients are without problems. It occurs when you are with patients and members of our *team*. The sacred times cause you to remember why you became a nurse in the first place. And, they inspire you when you're not experiencing the ideal.

My cohort of nursing friends at DG knew that at a more privileged hospital—serving more privileged patients—we would never have acquired the skills that made us the crackerjack nurses we all turned out to be. We never would have encountered so many opportunities or dealt with so many patient emergencies, which allowed us to make independent life-and-death decisions. We were creating a new reality of nursing care.

Today, standing orders exist because of the early efforts of nurses like us, who started IVs, sent labs, gave meds, determined which patients should be seen right now by a physician and which ones could wait—sometimes for hours. All of the actions we initiated with patients were based on what had become excellent assessment skills. We also felt empowered to say "no" to a physician's order to discharge a patient if we didn't think the patient was ready to leave. Or, to insist a doctor leave caring for one patient and come in and work with us when we knew that the patient we were with had a greater potential to have a worse outcome.

Nurses made decisions, often in the middle of the night or in the early morning hours, and when we looked back and saw that our decisions had saved a life. We and the medical staff, gained more confidence that the direction we were moving was safe and improved the care that the patients received. This was not done clandestinely; it evolved with much thought and was then communicated to other nurses at conferences, in published articles, and with our own research that we initiated.

We worked with nursing leadership, with advance practice nurses, while reading and speaking with PhD nurses to gain their expertise and perspectives of how to best gather information, pilot programs and report our clinical findings statistically and in together we validated our innovative ideas with other nurses. We began to publish; *first* articles and then we submitted our own research findings to nursing organizations for publication.

Our worth wasn't measured in tasks alone.

- We grew in our understanding of how difficult life can be for some people through no fault of their own.
- We learned what compassion and forgiveness really meant, and how powerful they were.
- We learned that "control" and what we did, made a difference, but not always.
- We learned that judging people whose lives we could only experience from the outside looking in would never justify what society agreed was a violation of our established humanness.
- We learned to provide hope, to be honest, to advocate, and to be silent when appropriate.
- We learned to use every bit of our education, expertise and skills to improve patient outcomes.

As astounding as the last bulleted statement sounds, I do not remember one patient error committed by a registered nurse!

Errors must have been made, but there was never a case brought up in our RN, MD, joint educational forums (or in private conversations) where there were any cases of bad judgment that resulted in a bad patient outcome.

We grew as professionals; we grew as people. We had the opportunity to take these valuable clinical and life lessons and apply them to our own lives outside of the hospital. We learned team skills and had opportunities to *be there* for each other. We all were essential.

Not having to prove yourself or the value of the tasks you performed provided the backdrop for innovative, conscious risk taking. It took away sniping at each other and any feelings of not being respected. We had "power" arguments, but I think most of us remember them as being centered on issues of communication and how to handle necessary differences of opinions when our roles were expanding and consistency in care delivery was needed.

Freedom. Power. Strength. Respect. These ingredients create an ideal environment for a human being to become his or her best self. Environments with these characteristics set forth the opportunity both as individuals and as a group to create very real visions. These environmental factors coupled with the need to improve care and outcomes encouraged innovative, collegial approaches to improve the care patients communicated that they wanted in support of their health and healing journeys.

Nurses in highly diverse settings recognize that new frontiers in health care exist locally in the communities where they live and in faraway war-torn countries. Places where lawlessness has such a strong hold on the country that a foreseeable peace is not yet on the horizon, and in places with diseases for which treatments are not yet relevant because resources can't surmount gargantuan geographical or political barriers, or in places where the populations needing help have exhausted what others before us could not sustain in delivering.

These frontiers must also include supporting patients who are never going to "get it right." Patients that we as caregivers often complain about as being the cause of their own problems. And this list must include places where we as nurses are also still struggling to "get it right." In other words, *Nursing Camelots* exist in many places and are waiting for each of *us* to be a part of turning dark places into *shining moments.*

New nurse-led models with expanded nursing responsibilities and skills are now being actualized and delivered that are very autonomous and fill unmet healthcare needs of individuals and populations as a whole. With the expansion and re-defining of one team member's skills, knowledge and behaviors, a cascade of change is set in motion that results in all team members' roles changing. A great deal of resistance is avoided when the planning and implementation of these tasks, role relationships and desired outcomes do not come only from the top down.

Irene had no words but her body spoke to me

How will you know that it's time to move on in a job, I was once asked. I said I didn't know at that time. I was just about to find out how I did know exactly when it was time to go. Having Ainsley, marrying Bruce, all were storybook perfect, but they put me into a different situation. I was responsible for a beautiful baby girl. My husband depended on me; together, we made a family. I wasn't the happy-go-lucky girl without any ties anymore. I couldn't be carefree about my safety or my future any longer.

At least that was my ostensible reason for leaving, but there was one incident at DG that pushed me to a limit of which even I wasn't aware. One patient experience was just too painful for me to continue working there.

I had been a mom for not quite a year the night in April of 1987 when I worked the 5:00 p.m. to 3:00 a.m. shift. Halfway through the shift, a couple came in with a little girl who looked shockingly like my little Ainsley: petite in structure, with white-blonde hair and big gorgeous, lashed eyes. This little girl, held by her father, made me smile as I walked up to this young family.

I smiled at the tiny stranger, but the little girl didn't move or smile back. She seemed to get smaller by the minute, curling up tighter into herself.

Hmm, I said to myself, she should be past the stranger anxiety stage. She seemed to be so distant and ... alone. My smile vanished, and the hair on the back of my neck felt tingly. Why didn't she turn to her mother or father for comfort, I wondered?

"Why are you here with your little girl tonight?" I asked the couple, noticing that neither of them had offered any physical expression or eye movements to indicate they were pulled in by *something* in their little girl's fawn-eyed, detached manner. The parents stood close to each other, but no sense of closeness or warmth emanated from them to each other or to their daughter. I found it difficult to take my eyes away from the little girl.

Waiting for their answer, my own mind went into high alert. I saw that they had not brought in anything—a bottle, a comfort blanket, a toy—with them. *Something is not right with this baby girl and her parents* my senses were telling me, yet I kept my face expressionless as I walked them back to an available room just steps away.

Something is not right with this baby girl and her parents.

Usually, I would have put a child at the end of the hall where the pediatric patients were placed, but not this one. I wanted to make sure she would not be taken from the ER until I knew she was safe.

After entering the room, I asked again, "What brings you here tonight?"

"It's her—she's not walking right," the father said.

"She looks very young," I said. "How old is she?"

"Old enough to be walking," the father said.

I looked at the mother, who hadn't said a word. Her face was not blank, just so veiled that I hoped that my eyes, facial expression, and body language were encouraging. I wanted her to know that I could wait till she was ready to risk saying something, or for her eyes to dart over to her daughter to tell me that she loved her little girl. Maybe not yet, but it will come, I thought as my gaze returned to the child who needed to have a name so that I didn't do what I sensed I was doing and that was to think of her as Ainsley.

"How old is old enough?" I asked, my sense of dread accelerating.

Just then, the little girl began to moan. She didn't turn to her mother or father for comfort. She just mewed.

"What do you think is going on?" I asked.

"I've tried to teach her to walk and to talk," the father snorted. "My wife gave up trying."

Finally, the wife spoke up. "She's not stupid like you say," she said to her husband. "She's just too little to walk, and she does talk to me," she bravely squeaked before looking back to the floor.

That was the only comment I would hear this woman make. The man didn't turn his head when his wife spoke. He didn't look at his daughter either as she moaned. He put all of his energy into challenging me with his unblinking, glaring, dark eyes as if to assess my compliance with his "eye fuck" demeanor. I knew this look; I had encountered it before.

"Do you think your daughter is stupid?" I asked the man, encouraging my voice to remain calm. I looked down at the little girl, who I thought I saw glance furtively upward toward her mother or possibly at me.

"Something's not right with her. And now she won't even try to walk," he said, as he placed the little girl on the exam table. He did it in such a way that showed he felt she was much too heavy for him to hold any longer. The child couldn't have weighed more than 12 pounds.

I looked at the mother and the little girl, hoping to communicate warmth and safety in my eyes, but they didn't receive the message. The mother looked down at the floor, and so did her child. Both were silent.

A medical assistant was passing the cubicle at that moment, and he saw my worried glance and noticed we were in an unusual room for a pediatric consult. A minute later, smart professional that he was, he returned with a stuffed animal, a little kitten, which he held out to see if her parents or I would take it from him to give to the little girl.

"How old is she, exactly?" I asked the parents, holding out the little stuffed kitten for the child to make even a small movement toward.

"She's a year old, old enough to be walking and not carried like a baby," the father said authoritatively, as if he were addressing a roomful of ignorant people.

"What is her name?" I asked as I slowly advanced my hands toward her to just take a safe check of her pulse at her wrist.

"I'd like to take her vital signs," I told them. What I wanted to do was cuddle this little waif, but I was aware that possibly any touch would be perceived fearfully and result in her going to a place still deeper inside of herself that had provided safety in the past.

I again asked, "And what is your beautiful little girl's name?" looking at the mother, who also seemed to be becoming smaller and more invisible.

The father spoke up. "Irene," he said.

It was as if this child's needs were completely ignored. Possibly in their haste to come to the hospital, in their worry over little Irene, I cautioned myself to consider, neither parent knew what to do. When I picked up hostility from them, I considered that possibly they also had been treated this way in the past. In an effort not to rush and give the impression that this environment could become more than just hostile, quickly, depending on what the father said and how Irene presented when she was examined, we all held our collective breath. I had a suspicious story and an extremely vulnerable patient, but in this suspended time frame when an abused child is brought in and the realization that the victim would be separated from her abuser is being made, it was easy to shift my attention back to Irene. Irene lay quietly on the exam table as if she were used to going along with other people's plans for her. It was not until I gently touched her leg that she cried out with obvious physical pain.

Neither parent moved or said a thing. I looked at the child again, at her legs. Now I noticed with quiet horror that both of her legs were not just thin but angulated in a manner that suggested they might have been broken.

I didn't say anything. My heart was beating hard. I kept an arm on the little girl's arm, instinctively stroking it with my thumb. I wanted to protect her from the trauma that had already, I feared, occurred.

"Um, I tried to teach her to walk," the father said hurriedly, "before her legs got bad."

"Get me a warm blanket," I called to the young medical assistant hovering outside the door, "and the senior resident, please; ask him to come here."

Then I turned to the father. "How did you try to teach her to walk?" I asked, hoping my voice wouldn't shake.

"Well, I held her up under her arms, you know, over and over," he said. "I did it over a bed, then the floor, and let her go. Like you teach a dog to swim, you toss them into the water and they learn fast enough," he added self-righteously.

I felt anger and disgust when I hiked up her little nightie to look at her legs, but that feeling didn't even compare to the turmoil inside me when this man explained what he'd done, why, and ended with, "It's not my fault she's slow." To my complete amazement he didn't try to lie or con me. Why should he, I realized. He was a supremely confident, angry man who molded the world of his wife and daughter into his reality because he had gotten away with it. Striding into the ER, complaining about his noncompliant one-year-old daughter.

When the senior resident arrived, I asked the father to repeat why they brought their daughter in to be seen. As he did, the doctor and I looked at each other.

This was abuse of a different order than we were used to seeing, the parents not hiding it, lying, or denying any responsibility for their child being injured. I had seen plenty of perpetrators of violent abuse blame their victims like Irene's father did. I had experienced adults blaming crying babies for their hurting someone else or their "stupid" kids being the cause of them doing something mean, hurtful, or dangerous. However, this man continued to be convinced that he needed "someone that knows how to train a kid, not the two of you who know nothing about kids thinking that I've done something wrong." He had correctly picked up that we did not agree with him that his daughter was stupid or that "if it's good enough to train a dog this way, then it's good enough for a kid."

The X-rays came back faster than they normally would, led me to believe that Anne, another nurse on duty that night had radiology shoot and deliver the results in record time.

We knew we would find injuries. There were, in fact, recent fractures in both of Irene's upper legs and also in the smaller bones of her lower legs. What made all of us gasp was the number of healing fractures in both of her upper and lower legs, too many to count without a magnifying glass—and one small fracture in one wrist, as if to defend herself one last time before she gave up.

Placing the tiny stuffed kitten with Irene under the warmed blanket I had placed on her, I stayed in the room while the doctor *invited* the parents to go with him to see her X-rays. As soon as they left, so did we. To safety, a back office where her parents would not be able to find their daughter. Irene had totally covered herself with the blanket and as I walked away with her possibly too snuggled up to my body, telling her what a wonderful little girl she was and that she would not be hurt by us, she fell asleep.

When Social Services and the police arrived, the physician examining Irene's films informed them Irene would not be going home with them tonight; she needed to be admitted because of all of her injuries. The father still did not sense any threat to himself, but the physician informed him that he and his wife were going to be charged with reckless endangerment of a child. The father said he was "shocked" that anyone thought he had broken "any laws." He was arrested, and so was his wife.

Irene did not cry. She was safe under the warm blanket, covered, invisible. I handed her to the social worker, and when I went back to see them after the parents were taken to the county jail, Irene peeked above her blanket as she sipped apple juice. No tears, no fear, no outward expression of any emotion. I had to believe that she at least felt safe, and that maybe she felt deep inside a warmth, a connection with someone who was not going to harm her.

I had confidence that the legal system would take care of things, but I didn't know what to do with the rage inside me. I had cried tears before over patients. I had talked with other nurses about patients I couldn't take my mind off of; I had identified and worked through many experiences with patients before that made me feel angry or powerless through the years. I would do this again, and it would "work," I was sure, but I didn't want to talk to anyone now. This patient, this little Irene, was different. I went up to see her the next day, but she had already been transferred to Children's Hospital. I never saw her again, but I'll never forget her.

I thought I knew how to get over it; I was "good" at working through tough patient experiences, but somehow, this last instance of abuse was too much. I went about the business of caring for patients, but when I was at home with Ainsley and Bruce, I couldn't reveal the pain I felt, and I couldn't suppress it any longer.

After witnessing so many problems over the years and helping to solve many of them—noticing and reporting, appearing in court, testifying—I now doubted my effectiveness. After being with this little girl, even when I wasn't thinking about her I was always carrying her with me, clutching her to me, away from everyone, everything else in *our* world. I hoped somehow the pain I felt for her was keeping her safe and alive. That didn't make sense, but neither did harming a little girl, asking her to do the impossible. I didn't want to think about this little girl, or the others like her, anymore—not right now, not when I had to have my heart open for my own little girl.

A month later, I turned in my resignation. "Wow, Julie, are you really leaving the ER?" I heard wherever I went. "Why?"

"Because I want to stay home with Ainsley. I'll probably be back, but who knows. There is this great job (*escape*, I think I even said once) as a nursing supervisor that I think I'll apply for," I'd answer as my voice trailed off and my back was to the person to whom

I had been talking, feeling like I was still falling farther down, down, down to some unknown, unfamiliar down-under place.

There hadn't been a position as a house supervisor, but then suddenly one opened up. There were also changes happening at home. Bruce had been accepted into medical school. We needed the income, and I needed to support our family, but I couldn't any longer, here. Leaving became easy and desirable.

I was leaving *this* Camelot, although a month ago I could not have even imagined leaving. But that was before Irene. Now I had to.

My years as a nurse in the emergency room at Denver General was an extraordinary time in my career. *We* didn't get cold, mean, or uncaring. *We* didn't get hardened at all. *We* became more sensitive to life's pain, victims' pain, perpetrators' pain, and my own pain. Ultimately, our group of nurses from the last decade began to leave.

Marion left because she said, "I can't be the wife and mom that I want to be working here, and now I am choosing my family." Fun loving Anne left when she met the man that "exceeded all of my dreams and we plan on having a houseful of boys and we're getting started now." Cathy left to pursue her PhD in Nursing. Several others left because of a painful break up or because of a painful patient experience that we didn't all know about until our reunion in 2009. Each of us responded to a stimulus that told us that it was time to move on.

After leaving Denver General, I took a three year research position at Maricopa Medical Center Emergency Medicine Residency Program where my husband was completing his medical education in Emergency Medicine. Participating in supporting the varied topics the residents investigated gave me a strong understanding of the role of identifying pertinent problems to be studied and how answers could be achieved by selecting the most appropriate research methods and statistical testing—all of which advanced the specialty of emergency care.

I then worked for a major pharmaceutical company to educate and advertise the use of the new 2A 3B platelet inhibitors. This was eye-opening and financially very lucrative, but I found this traveling position difficult as the mother of two young teenagers. This move into the for-profit world did lead me to start a business with a fellow nurse when we returned to Colorado.

Developing a business plan and bringing into reality a company that assisted seniors to remain in their own homes (after entering into an emergency department due to an injury or change in their physical or mental status) was difficult every day for the first year we were in business. It evoked feelings of being overwhelmed just as I had experienced in every new position I took. This was not daunting now; this was vitalizing.

Each of the positions, in their own ways had aspects of perfection, growth and ah-ha moments. They each presented challenges that I had not faced before, but I had the confidence that the unknowns could be successfully mastered. I believed that I could re-create successes in nursing as I changed jobs and believed that the problems I encountered were only hurdles that actually seemed to make each work environment more interesting. I applied lessons from each place I had worked.

Live your questions now,
and perhaps even without knowing it,
you will live along some distant day
into your answers.

—RAINER MARIA RILKE

CHAPTER 16

Shock, Anger, Disappointment: Once Again, Didn't I Think That I Knew It All?

I was working in a place where we hadn't been successful at bringing about a more collaborative, respectful, and values-driven environment for reasons that took years longer for me to discover.

> *"Nursing is a noble profession*
> *but too often a terrible job.*
> *I love nursing but ..."*
> —DANIEL F. CHAMBLISS, author

"Honey, are you sure you want to go back and be a bedside nurse?" my husband asked, with an amused, look-like-you're-listening expression on his kind face.

"Mom, you do everything fast except ski," said Braden, our 13 year old, with his adoring eyes, "but do you really think you can do all of the work?"

"Why?" asked Ainsley, our 16-year-old future physician. It was more of a statement than a question.

This family conference was a spontaneous expression of confusion on their part, and truth to tell I didn't have all the answers either. Why indeed had I, at age 53, decided to go back to work at an Ambulatory Care Clinic? I was going back to "bedside nursing" because simply, I missed it. I wanted to be in the trenches again. I wanted to feel that excitement, that one-on-one intimacy that came so easily and satisfactorily, between me and my patients. I wanted to feel nursing through my fingers, my hands, my heart, once again.

However, my happy return did not work out exactly as planned.

Lulu, the last nurse to leave DG, had guided me to this new job. "After DG, this place will be a cinch for you," she said. I planned to work per diem, to work for fun, to pay for some extras in my home life. I was going to be a "refrigerator nurse." My life was full and I specifically planned on not getting involved in the politics of my new workplace.

"I'm only buying one set of scrubs," I told friends. "Because I don't think I'll be staying that long." And true to my intent, I laid low for six months. I was quiet; I asked a lot of questions. It took me awhile to understand a union environment that had its own hierarchy of staff and access to information. It added another layer of decision making that often seemed to pit labor against management, hindering the partnership that it was designed to enhance.

Six months after arriving at the clinic, having received no formal orientation, I asked our nurse manager for an organizational chart. This system had a trailblazing electronic medical record and had as its focus, preventative health activities that were very integrated between primary care and all of the specialties that patients needed. But I couldn't find nursing procedures that were appropriate for the level of detail that we as an urgent care clinic needed.

"The nurse manager's management style is to treat us all like we are her extended family of six daughters who often squabble," remarked a senior nurse as she commented "and nursing seems like we are an afterthought to management," she calmly told me. "Try not to care so much," she advised.

But "not caring" is simply not in my intellectual vocabulary. It had been through *caring a lot* that all of the positive changes in my previous work sites had resulted in tremendous site specific gains. Changes in systems and changes in personnel competencies occur because there is the belief that improvements can be realized. I requested a meeting with the next nurse manager that took over the clinic, stating, "I find it difficult to perform my duties because of the inadequate number of nebulizer machines, and the lack of an ice machine or fluid/blanket warmer which creates inefficient and very basic care and comfort deficiencies."

No response to *that* memo. I stopped the head nurse in the hall. "Hey, did you get my memo? I was hoping to help you procure those items because the MDs, RNs and support staff all said they'd been complaining for a long time about those two issues."

"I know about those needs," she remarked. Shortly afterward, she took another position in the organization.

Five years, three nurse managers and many staff meetings later, we as a staff requested an intermediary, a consultant, someone to assist us in having our concerns heard. It was as if the revolving door of hiring nurse managers by the highest level of nursing leadership seemed to hire managers that couldn't manage, problem-solve or have their voices heard by the Director levels of Nursing.

Endless variations in staff meetings and in one-to-one conversations now sounded like "just complaining" to us as well. How to elevate our needs from being viewed as just grumbling or being negative by our nursing leaders became difficult when I realized that we, the nursing staff, were perceived as the problem, not a source of contributing to improved care.

From my fifth to tenth year of working in this clinic, we had another three nurse managers. We asked for and got a designation as a self-managed clinic but with all levels of staff MDs, Physician Assistants, Nurse Practitioners, RNs, and our support staff reporting to their own department heads, any strong functioning as a cohesive team remained out of reach.

Administrators who believe that all types of nursing care are so similar that one RN can be substituted with any other RN if the need arises, creates potentially very unsafe and inefficient patient care conditions.

Within all of the clinical sites in our organization, some sites were happy with how they delivered care while others felt ignored. We met with other RNs, feeling confident that if our numbers increased as a staff and the patients we collectively served, then our nursing leaders would hear our needs.

Training subtly replaced education and nowhere was this more obvious than with the Ebola scare in 2013. My nurse manager came up to me when I was triaging 22 patients in the opening hour of the clinic. He sat beside me asking me to "just check off these five boxes to indicate that you have been instructed as to how to care for suspected possible victims."

"How many hours of education did you have on this?" I asked when he stated that he really had to leave by 6:30 this evening, even as our clinic had just opened thirty minutes ago at 6 p.m.

Groaning, he replied, "Ten long hours." "Really" I said, "you will not be having any direct patient contact but we the RN staff will be the first line for any suspected Ebola patients and I get five continuously interrupted minutes to sign a paper that states that I received Ebola training?"

If a job is measured in minute to minute satisfaction, I have had many golden moments. In this position, at the end of the shift, five to ten minutes were needed from one of the RNs to sort through the various trash containers to separate out any discarded trash that might have a patient identifier on it to insure patient privacy. We "proved" that as RNs we did not consider going through the trash, or leaving the clinic to take a urine specimen to the lab (or to clean up the floors if someone vomited on them because housekeeping was not available) as tasks that we were "too good" to do. These moments created wasted minutes.

This was an "egalitarian" place to work; lots of people did lots of other people's work. I might be pushing my patient to X-ray as the medical assistant was asking another patient vague, rote questions about his or her chest pain. The RN staff attempted to bring up prioritizing tasks based on education and experience of our team members, but who did what changed from shift to shift depending on who was on.

The division widens

The distance between "us and them" ... clinical staff and management, widened. Courageous conversations, unit-based team goal-setting, and hit-or-miss staff meetings ended with platitudes of 'thanks for the great job you all come in and do every day.' This soon resulted in meetings being canceled two months in advance.

Administrators who believe that all types of nursing care are so similar that one RN can be substituted with any other RN if the need arises, create potentially very unsafe and inefficient patient care conditions. If a nurse has never worked with babies and children, then the belief that these patients are just "small adults," or that a pregnant woman is just a "patient and a half," is dangerous. When a non-nursing administrator believes this, then it is the responsibility of nursing leadership to communicate that this belief does not promote safe care.

The belief that "clinic patients" are not as critical as ICU/ER patients is a convenience for those persons seeking to find the most versatile and least expensive level of staff to provide care. Clinic patients in our setting had major cardiac, obstetrical, neurological and trauma concerns. They needed to be triaged and cared for by experienced staff.

Throughout all of my years in nursing, I have witnessed extreme flexibility of nurses stepping up and doing what was needed to deliver competent, safe care. That is the expectation of what nurses *do*. Advocating for safer care is also what good nurses do. But there is a limit to flexibility.

"How can I provide you the information you need to make increasingly unsafe working conditions less so?" I asked several nurse managers over the years. "Who can I go to, to have our issues heard? Who do *you* go to when you have a nursing issue, a staffing issue, or a problem that you can't solve" These and many other documented, politely worded concerns, questions, and attempts to reach out were met with silence.

Did I not possess the moral courage, resilience, or skills to take pragmatic information and actualize it into transformative behavior, I asked myself? I had been successful at being part of a team that had gathered information, articulated it successfully and then worked through the channels of having needs collaboratively resolved in the past, but not here.

Talking with other staff members about our problems was cathartic enough to diffuse the anger and frustration that became the pervasive feel of this clinic. If you had a good or great shift, then it buoyed you up to keep coming back. If you had an unsafe, chaotic, and personally unfulfilling shift, where you were not happy with the care you were able to give, you walked out at the end of the shift and denied that it was *that bad.*

Then in 2013, what should have been a desired occurrence for any healthcare site occurred: the number of patients who selected our clinic as the place to receive their care grew beyond anyone's projections. The Affordable Care Act (ACA) provided health care to millions of persons that had previously been unable to access care, for years in some cases. Healthcare concerns neglected because of cost, accessibility, and more pressing life issues brought in many new patients. Forecasting had underestimated the increase in numbers, but as the patients arrived, we believed that this deluge of new patients in all of our sites would result in changes that had been neglected, but couldn't be ignored any longer.

Staff satisfaction surveys were conducted as mandated by NCQA (the National Committee for Quality Assurance), but the results were not shared with staff. HEDIS measurements (important for healthcare organizations to receive favorable press and payment by governmental programs such as Medicare and Medicaid) became the barometers of whether care was good enough, since staff input was ignored.

Now it was even worse that all of the equipment had been placed for the convenience of the person ordering the equipment (by consecutive numbers, not by use patterns) or that the "just-in-time" ordering meant we often ran out of medium crutches or laceration-repair sterile trays after a busy warm weather weekend, or that nurses were not replaced because of overtime costs never budgeted (the budget still has never been shared with the staff even after twelve years of requesting this information).

The agreed-upon number of RNs on duty was four. This dropped to three, and then it slowly dropped "occasionally" to two on Saturdays and Sundays (our busiest shifts because only the ER was open on weekends for patients in this healthcare network). Staff members did indeed work harder, as predicted by management. They also worked less safely. Incident reports, especially regarding medication errors, increased.

In 2015 we received a memo stating, "All staffs are to take a one-hour lunch break in a shift lasting more than five hours. This is a federal law, and the institution could be fined if this rule is not adhered to." Staff members increasingly called and wrote the nurse manager, stating that meeting the requirements of this memo would place the clinic and all of the patients and staff at risk. "I'm sorry, I'm doing the best I can," he pleaded with us to understand.

Nurses feeling trapped, powerless, and devalued was new for me but was not new to the profession historically.

Not taking a lunch also resulted in overtime and that was unacceptable. Somehow, this made sense to him that overtime should be more important than leaving one RN in a clinic with twenty-four rooms for two hours during every busy twelve hour Saturday and Sunday. We found his lack of not being alarmed by this time, not surprising. Ultimately, we didn't take lunches when there were only two RNs on and it didn't seem to make a difference to anyone.

Our union representative did all that she could do to high-light our concerns. Physicians knew of the staffing shortage and unsafe environment in which our care was often delivered, but they along with us were told to just wait, we are "re-designing the delivery of our care." We continued to collect anecdotal information that was not trusted as being accurate. We asked for an in-depth site visit to take place, or a consultant to come and address our issues, for the last five years. This organization that had many, many consultants come in and provide communication, leadership and team building presentations to them, could not find the budget to provide this for the employees they managed.

I called our state Board of Nursing, which allowed for anonymous questioning, to seek guidance as to how to deal with our unsafe staffing situation. *Could a case of abandonment of the patient be used to demonstrate the need for safer staffing?* I asked in writing. "Staffing is not an issue for a state board of nursing to involve itself with," the director of clinical issues responded back to me.

"Julie, you can afford to be fired, but I can't. Thanks for speaking up about unsafe practices, but we can do the job they are telling us to do because that's what nurses do—we get tough when the situation requires us to be tough."

"I don't think this is what our education and our experience has taught us to believe in 2015," I texted and shared verbally.

Where to go now? I asked myself. After choosing to stay this long, I didn't want to walk away yet.

Nurses feeling trapped, powerless, and devalued was new for me but was not new to the profession historically.

Were my issues important, or were they only relevant to those of us practicing in this type of setting? What was I expecting other nurses in other sites to do about the fact that we still hadn't been able "to get it right"? I was working in a place where we hadn't been successful at bringing about more substantive changes, only those that looked good on paper. "It's as if the filters of acceptability of "no lawsuits, no bad deaths, and good HEDIS (Health Effectiveness Data and Information Set) measurements, which are publicly available pieces of marketing information, were all that seemed to matter."

For the first time, I was not able to be a part of improving a clinical nursing dilemma of articulating what nurses needed and why. We as a staff continued to look to outside nursing resources for guidance. We believed the mission statement of where we worked: "to place the patient at the center of the care we deliver." Skilled, savvy, sophisticated, mutually advanced problem resolution skills, communication and problem solving techniques, were not utilized because this required some interest, some cooperation, and we were unable to capture anyone's concern. We had fallen between the cracks of primary and emergent care that functioned well.

I looked to literature and to my academic colleagues from within nursing and external to my organization to find any applicable perspectives to which I was blind to or of which I was unaware. Variations of "You have to have leadership that backs you for any change to occur and if the status quo appears to be working for them, then change will not occur," was what I repeatedly was told.

This type of impasse had occurred to nurses *in the past*, I knew. The number of patients we saw in our clinic was approximately three hundred patients a week, too many to ignore if these patients are the ones that you serve. Too many to give up on we all continued to believe.

I had never been fully aware of the causes and depth of nursing dissatisfaction until this last decade. Being frustrated, disillusioned and then angry over a long period of time is well established as being at the root of nursing moral decay. Knowing that I was not alone, but getting fatigued trying to find someone that was accountable, led me to return once again to school.

All of the events over the last decade could have been intervened upon by our nursing leadership inviting and encouraging dialogues of discontent. By not providing this opportunity, we attempted other ways to circumvent the lack of response that our assessments and recommendations did not activate.

But there were only so many "work-arounds" that we could put into place. Discontent increases behaviors that are detrimental to the employee and to patients receiving care. We were frustrated and angry, but our disillusionment brought us together as a team. What resulted was that we believed that our patients trusted and expected us to give them good care just because we were *doctors and nurses.* We apologized often for slowness, or not keeping them informed. The power of taking scraps of time to give a hastily worded, quick popping of our heads in their rooms, to say, "You haven't been forgotten. I think it will be another ten minutes on your labs. Are you doing OK?" was sometimes the most caring action we took on some shifts.

Giving in would have been easy, persevering required tenacity, professionalism and reflected our staff of twelve's belief that this is what patients expected of us each time they came in to be seen.

Why are you looking for your car keys
at night, under a street light,
when you know you didn't lose them here?

—JIM KENESER, economist, 2014

CHAPTER 17

Looking Back to Move Forward

Conference titles such as: *Authentic Leadership;*
Circling Back on Old Problems; Not Just a Nurse;
Compassion, Fatigue and Burnout; The Dilemma
with the Nurse Manager Role are topics by
nursing leader Rose Sherman, EdD, RN, FAAN,
which leads one to be confident that there are practice
issues that maybe should be behind us, but are not.

We are made wise not by the recollection
of our past but by the responsibility of the future.
—GEORGE BERNARD SHAW, author

fascinating conversation that occurs frequently in my life with nursing colleagues and random strangers goes like this. I ask, "What was your experience like when you were in the hospital 20 (or 30 or 40) years ago?" and the response comes back invariably: "I felt more cared for."

Fascination enters in because 20 years ago—to say nothing of 30 or 40 years ago—we knew a lot less. Twenty plus years ago, patients died of conditions that are preventable today (pneumonia; wound infections; the effects of long periods of inactivity; the wrong kind of IV fluids). Yet the responders to my question never mention unsafe care or an untimely death.

It is not that their expectations were lower in the past or that they were naïve. It is simply that they felt more cared for.

Care—addressing a patient's needs—is the primary focus of nursing.

I realized that "historically" nursing could now be referenced from two perspectives: in reference to Florence Nightingale, and to my own *history*. The site specific problems I had experienced in my career I realized were not isolated to only "my world" of nursing. Reviewing my complete history of places and people who had redefined and redesigned how nursing care was delivered, I chose to believe that even with inertia that had been in place a long time, things could change.

Florence Nightingale resurfaced as a role model to me now, for the second time in my life, since first learning about her in nursing school almost 50 years ago. Historically, a great deal is known about Nightingale through her prolific writings. The most original and important nursing educational tenet that she felt was pivotal to developing the specialty of nursing was only *partially* followed through with her arrival to America in 1873 to Belleview Hospital in New York. She recognized that nursing was a unique body of knowledge and skills and defined what these were. This belief was ingrained and transferred with her from England.

Nightingale believed that nursing education and practice be managed and supervised by nurses. "Patients," she believed, "received the best care when no single power is ascendant," for when this situation occurs, "there is a perpetual rub between who is put into the position of being subservient." Physicians and male dominated religious leaders had other ideas of who could best manage nurses: that nurses shouldn't be under the direction of nurses.

The use of the description of nurses as being "hand-maidens to physicians" remains today, and although dismissed by the majority of nurses and physicians as being a dated term, remnants of this concept remain.

The negative implications of this persona has unfortunately remained and is one of the reasons that there are nursing historians, theorists and educators who believe that she is not the most relevant or ideal person to highlight. Men today may feel more marginalized by Nightingale than women, but the irony is that we all are still affected by this moniker.

The *shift*: invisibility becomes a reality and mediocrity the new fear to battle against.

Ninety years ago, where and how nurses were educated was changing along with what other women were educationally demanding. Women sought access to university educations in professional fields that had previously been closed to them such as engineering, law and medicine. The second wave of feminism in the 1960s resulted in what should have been a wonderfully mutual, supportive relationship with nurses and non-nurses alike. It didn't happen.

Feminists fought hard for more educational, social, sexual and financial advancement that resulted in the most transformational shift in the lives of women ever in the history of humankind. In fighting for equality in educational arenas, women demanded that they be given the opportunity to compete educationally which would then allow them access to previously restricted, higher-paying professional occupations. As entrance into the best schools became a reality, so did acceptance into medical schools. This was wonderful, but there was one unforeseen casualty, and that was nursing. As medical school enrollment went up, many women asked: Why be a nurse *if* I could be a doctor?

For those of us on the last tide going out of wanting to be nurses, the riptide created by those nurses who felt that being a doctor was "better than" being a nurse was awkward. The paradox then became, and remains today, that feminists fought for the choice "to be what you wanted to be," with gender not being a determinant, but for those women who chose to be nurses, it was seen as being a second tier choice. Nursing is still seen in the eyes of many as being "like medicine, just less than."

If patient needs haven't changed from wanting competent, compassionate care, then what occurred that made patients begin to feel that they needed to have a family member present with them if they became hospitalized, a common belief and practice today?

Nurses consistently are rated as the most trustworthy of professionals, yet something caused a shift in patient confidence with the care they were receiving. As the front line of patient contact, the nurse was often the person perceived as either the person that caused a mistake to occur, or should have done something to prevent a complication from occurring. Simultaneously occurring was the prioritization of patient safety as the delivery of care became increasingly more complex. Healthcare organizations are in the business of financing the care provided, with their bottom lines being scrutinized at a time when balancing explosive and expensive technological demands hit healthcare delivery like never before.

From my own "historical" perspective, clinical staffs are well aware of the challenge to provide increasingly complex care, yet keep costs down. The desire to quantify the tasks performed in relation to health outcomes that produce measurable positive health benefits to patients is also not new. What is also not new is that procedures, process, previous job descriptions and how care will be delivered—are all changing. Change is not new to those of us in health care. But the rate and degree of change is new.

The need to work collaboratively is also not new. The time frame to create and put into place new and altered systems and the staffs needed to deliver care differently is new and has created pressure on all of us. We do have to prove ourselves, our value, and I would also include, our visibility. Visibility in our own organizations and collectively to the public is needed.

Nursing leaders have been highly successful in many environments by being actively involved in brainstorming, decision making and budgeting for new ideas to transform care. The ability of leadership to recognize when changes are needed and to enlist input from the nurses they represent, results in successful outcomes. Conversely, nursing leaders that have not challenged themselves to explore and create new paths will in all likelihood not do so in the staffs they represent. The risk of not seeking innovation in others will result in stagnant mediocrity of care.

Task shifting, training replacing education, "enhanced job roles" and the "dumbing down" of what nurses provide to a task-only level is happening now. Hiring paramedics or non-RNs to work in critical care areas may appear to solve staffing financial challenges. *Hiring down*, or focusing on the care of patients from a task only perspective, when the delivery of health care demands a more educated work force is dangerous.

"What does a registered nurse do that is different from an LPN who costs less to educate and employ?" is a question I hear more now than five years ago. The risk of replacing RNs with LPNs as a cost effective alternative is very much a threat to patients, and yes, to the profession of nursing. The public rarely knows that an LPN's education is far less than an RN's. Yet, we are all valuable to patient care.

Four years compared to one year of education delivers far more information, practical experience, mentorship and competency. The RN has been educated to take their assessments and apply a wider basis of decision making, involving many resources within and external to the site the patient enters seeking care. There are organizations that are venturing out and hiring LPNs and paramedics to work in their ERs. Viewing patient needs and care as being tasks requiring minimal judgment and decision making results in validating what most registered nurses believe is the cause of eroding patient confidence. Increasing numbers of patients feel less cared for and less safe.

Patients should not be placed in this conundrum.

It is well documented that poor communication and collaboration that is not substantive is a major cause of nurses not remaining in nursing. This is also a deterrent for those considering nursing as a career. When the same problems are brought up year after year, and there is minimal or no acknowledgment that the areas of concern are of any priority, then distrust and lack of engagement eventually results in nurses leaving their profession. Sociologist and ethicist, Daniel F. Chambliss states,

Nurses and their work reveal clearly to us how we over-look, ignore and undervalue the crucial daily routines of which life and death are built.

This invisibility of the value of professional nursing care is not just a feeling but a reality in some environments.

When there are failures in communication and collaboration, coupled with gender, power, and a social culture that believes that change is taking place, but staff does not, this creates a demoralizing state and devalues the contribution of nurses.

I think nursing leaders, academics, and practicing nurses would all say there is more work that we need to initiate and follow through on if we are to retain, much less expand as a profession. We need the efforts of our academic experts and those in leadership positions to keep their focus on the person delivering direct patient care.

There is a great deal of diversity in how nurses currently assess their work environments. Many practicing nurses assess their environments as great or good. Registered nurses who provide hands-on patient care and feel autonomous, respected, empowered, and are able to use their education and experience, do exist. However, many RNs do not believe that the organizations that employ them actually support their utilizing their education and experiences as optimally as they currently are.

I believe that in speaking out more publicly about the roadblocks and inability to move the care delivered by my colleagues and myself in our own organization—that I am giving voice to the invisibility of other nurses, and giving voice to nurses that do not want to give up and possibly leave nursing. We are all guardians of the trust the public has in us as nurses and any dissatisfaction with the care we deliver is valuable to our profession as a whole, because we represent care that we know should be better than it is.

I strongly believe that we as a collective body of nurses must be aware and provide support to those nurses who are not yet "making it." Making it being defined as having achieved the autonomy and respect to achieve collaborative outcomes based on the input of all of us that became educated to provide nursing care. Many institutions are watching those sites that are attempting to provide care using a less educated nursing work force, different staffing ratios and systems that have economically prioritized procedures and processes. Ignoring and discounting nursings' input about these detrimental actions is occurring now. The liability to each nurse has risen and this liability is not small.

Lawsuits, Deaths, and HEDIS measurements are important but they do not capture what patients want when they are ill. Attempting to balance overall budgets by decreasing the expense of utilizing registered nurses is short-sighted.

Empirical data exists that supports decreased staff and preparedness of nurses effects patient satisfaction and safety. It is the nurse at the bedside that is left accountable for meeting the desired goals of the organization. Leaders that believe that their employees want to be engaged and committed to the patients they serve set the stage for valuing diversity of opinions from them.

*Expose your ideas
to the risk of controversy.*

—THOMAS J. WATSON,
founder of IBM

CHAPTER 18

Fifty Years
What's New, What's Not

"Vocation – The place where your deep gladness
meets the world's deep needs."
—FREDERICK BUECHNER,
WISHFUL THINKING: A THEOLOGICAL ABC

*T*he biggest impact on the profession of nursing is exactly what has impacted all of us in the last fifty years. Technology. Just as the evolution of the spoken word (orality) was impacted by the written word (literacy) the technological discoveries of the last fifty years, continues to impress and affect all of us worldwide. The computer was introduced in the 1940s; its impact on the entire world exceeded the dreams envisioned by its inventors.

The efficiency, accuracy, speed and breadth of information that is now available is of enormous value to health care. All three of these evolutionary changes have had a profound effect on how humans think and interact. Prior to the written word, we kept information "in our heads." Shifting from conversing with one another to utilizing the computer to serve as the conduit of how we learn, share and apply the vast amounts of *new* information is now available to us. Who would have thought that today we would communicate with each other, sitting in the same room, texting instead of orally conversing?

"High Tech, Low Touch" is a phrase that we in healthcare are sensitive to in working with patients. Compassion, sensitivity, sympathy, tolerance and touching can often feel like they take a back seat to the end point of us finding the perfect answer or solution available to us via computers. There is no question that the information and efficiencies available to every discipline in health care has not resulted in healthier patient outcomes.

> Approximately five years ago, I realized that a change was occurring with parents of sick or injured children.

What has not changed over time is that health and wellness is not achieved by information alone.

Patients have expectations of receiving the *best* care. We know this because when we ourselves are in the role of being a patient, we want the *best* care available. And as patients, we want to feel cared for, especially when what we want and need is not answerable with information. Approximately five years ago, I realized that a change was occurring with parents of sick or injured children. Where and how patients found comfort, was beginning to change. Fewer favorite blankets or stuffed animals for babies and younger pediatric patients accompanied them. Parents were now pulling out their cell phones.

I think most of us when we first saw this change in *lovie* objects, inwardly thought, how lazy, how detrimental to their child's overall good would result, by their child being offered, and preferring, a computerized comfort item. It took me many observations to realize that these objects did provide comfort and diversion from the pain or scariness of our clinical world.

Pictures of family members, pets, short home videos, Disney movies and music had replaced a soft blanket, a stuffed bunny or teddy bear.

Was a low tech *blankee* better than a little high tech phone they could hold, play with, see and hear their family members being there with them? Didn't they get too much stimulation already from technology as it was, we often remarked to each other? Yet, these items did engage and sooth frightened children. I shifted away from judging these new items as being inferior when I noticed that parents did still touch, coo, make eye contact, talk to and cradle their children in an effort to protect and shield them from our painful and threatening environment.

> Nursing care is not at risk of being "computerized"... unless we under-value what we uniquely provide.

Information obtained from the Internet has not taken the place of family, friends and neighbors that traditionally had been the source of passing down knowing what to do with health care questions. The internet can be a replacement or an adjunct to knowing when to come in and what to do when you are once again home and in need for information that we may not have given you when you were being seen. Knowledgeable patients are less dependent on believing that we in health care have all of the answers. There is simply too much information and too little time to provide all of what patients, and those caring for them, might need or find useful to know.

This change in the dependent relationship of patients to care providers took some getting used to by patients and physicians alike at first. This challenged the long held hierarchical position of the doctor patient relationship of the past. With increased information available to patients, a shift in how patients and care providers interacted occurred. Achieving desired health outcomes became more of a partnership as opposed to the hierarchical position of the patriarchal past.

Change doesn't stop. For now, from the world's smallest computers (Micro Mote: "smart dust") to the fastest (Petaflop: one thousand trillion calculations per second), all of this *assistance* won't replace what nurses believe that patients want and need; and that is to not feel invisible, abandoned and not being seen as unique. We touch patients with a look or action that may not involve physical touching at all. The value of care provided by nurses can partially be substituted by technology, but not completely.

Nursing care is not at risk of being "computerized" unless we under-value what we uniquely provide. Resisting the "taskification" of nursing care by others in the belief that nursing care is quantifiable to tasks that can be accomplished by someone that focuses only on the endpoint of the task will result in the loss of a powerful component to healing.

Sociologist, Daniel Chambliss author of *Beyond **Caring:** Hospitals, **Nurses** and the Social Organization of Ethics,* states that we as a society undervalue *caring* as a characteristic in many professions. He states that this is most evident in the nursing profession. Providing *caring,* competent care is why many highly dedicated and talented people choose nursing. Not surprisingly it is why some leave if they feel powerless to meet this goal. We in the profession want this entering ideal to remain.

For myself, I found that I became more attentive and was less distracted by whatever environment I was in when I experienced each patient encounter as unique from the minute I walked into the room and said, "Hello, my name is Julie and I am your nurse today." I learned to feel confident, knowing that I was committed to providing care that *would* be of value to my patient. Developing this *knowing* and believing that it was sustainable came over time because it was something I wasn't directly taught.

Maybe this is because it is a mind and heart place that each nurse must find for his or herself. Being cared for, feeling cared for in conjunction with all of the technology available to us, was difficult at first for us to assimilate but now seems easier to interface. We need patients to inform us if our technology interferes or seems to be a substitute for them receiving the care they expected.

Once the storm is over you won't remember
how you made it through, how you survived.
But one thing is certain.
When you come out of the storm
you won't be the same person who walked in.
That's what the storm is all about.

—Haruki Murakami, Japanese novelist

PART IV

NOBILITY

"I gift you with the courage to be."

—JEAN HOUSTON, PhD

CHAPTER 19

Compassion and Forgiveness: The Path to Discovery

When you don't know what to do,
learn something new.
—WINNIE THE POOH

*I*n 2010 I returned to school.

"We use the external world as a means to learn, guide us, and provide feedback regarding what is ultimately an internal inquiry for finding the meaning and purpose of our own unique lives," I heard this and wrote it down when I found myself back in school to get an MA in Psychology. Looking for answers outside of my world, I exchanged the desire to get a PhD in nursing (even though that had been my plan in 1990 when I got my MSN) to now wanting to look for meaning to *issues* that felt bigger than my own nursing world. As people grow in their awareness of who they are, they also seem to grow in their mutual supportiveness of each other and then of strangers.

Possibly I thought, when first hearing this sentiment. The next two years opened up many different points of view. I soon learned many more diverse scopes of meaning in what it meant to care for patients.

We all carry wounds that cause us pain and suffering. We all make judgments of people and circumstances that initially support what we believe to be standards for ourselves and *should* also be applied to others. We judge others by our values of right and wrong, and these judgments separate "us" from "them." One day we realize that our initial view of patients as different from "us" does not feel right anymore. Instead of separating and focusing on our difference, the hope is that growing in our own awareness of how we fit in this world causes us to become more tolerant and supportive of people who live their lives differently.

I learned that we in health care often create distance from patients in order to feel safe from being like "them." This slowly results in a disconnect that often fuses into frustration and anger. Why? Because as we disconnect, we lose the primary meaning or reason that most of us entered health care and that *was to care.*

From the beginning of my nursing education, I was taught that as nurses we *give care; we give compassion.* Setting up the nurse-patient relationship as an *exchange,* we provide care and compassion and our patients thank us, get better, and leave happy.

But if they do not reciprocate in some desired way that results in us feeling valued and appreciated, we may question, *how much longer can I go on doing this type of work for patients that don't appreciate me?* The essence of a caring relationship is that it carries no judgments; it is a relationship where we don't need to prove to each other our worthiness. Relating to patients compassionately is more than a warm feeling; it is an acceptance of them just as they are.

Judgments have as their focus the differences between us. Maybe not at first, but over time these judgments of what is acceptable behavior and who is good or bad can erode the kindness and initial desire to be of service to another. The more we find ourselves "upset because … ," or "I'd be happy if …. ," the greater the likelihood that a personal judgment is going on within us. Coming to work and viewing some patients as deserving whatever painful circumstance has happened to them, or judging a patient as being less worthy of compassionate care prevents us from the joy we once believed was special about being a nurse.

Eugene Richards, in his book *The Knife and Gun Club,* has as one of his central themes that trauma and pain often do not end on the street; rather trauma, pain and suffering often continue into the emergency room from the streets. Richards' book remains controversial because of its graphic photographs, which he included to grab and hold onto his readers' attention. This extremely sensitive man found the photos he himself took as painful, but he chose not to soften what being in an inner-city trauma center was like.

Is the opposite of judging, forgiving? Forgiving others is not condoning actions of theirs that we have determined to be wrong in some way. Emergency Department staff and numerous other healthcare workers come into contact with many people who commit crimes. Interestingly, the act of forgiving someone carries with it an element of wrongdoing by someone. When I judged others, I set up a judging relationship of there being a victim, a rescuer, and a perpetrator. This often resulted in someone being judged and blamed. And with blame, punishment is often seen as being the right consequence.

Staunchly held beliefs can, over time, cause cynicism, coldness and result in care givers feeling downtrodden by those, "deadbeats, POS (pieces of shit), the dregs of society." We had lots of words to describe some of our patients' behaviors. But again, over time this also didn't feel right. Considering yourself *better* than someone already struggling felt ... bad.

Forgiveness exists on two levels: forgiveness of others for their actions and forgiveness of ourselves for our judgements. By accepting and forgiving others we have judged, we are not letting them *off of the hook* for unacceptable behavior. Perpetrators do go to jail and do get punished. Each time I have been able to let go of my own personal judgments of right and wrong, good and evil, it was easier to be focused on their healing and wellness.

Have you *lost your mind, gone soft* a fellow nurse once asked me when she saw me grab the hand of a patient that had driven drunk and had killed someone? The young man was being moved about, stuck with IVs and had a huge open fracture of his femur with one end of the bone poking out through his skin. Everything we did to him was excruciatingly painful. He was terrified. I grabbed his hand, made and held eye contact with him while telling him, "Hang on for thirty seconds longer; we know you hurt."

> Forgiveness exsists on two levels: forgiveness of others for their actions and forgiveness of ourselves for our judgement.

This simple act opened me up immediately to such an exquisite, deeper level of understanding of what compassion was. This young man did not evoke any negative feelings I might have experienced in my past; rather I just remember feeling very close to him. He knew that the cops were present in the room and that he was hated by most of the people present, but I'd like to believe that having someone consider you worthy *just as you are, at your lowest, worst moment,* has got to let in a glimmer of hope that you should not give up on yourself.

As a nurse, I have had many opportunities to recognize my own projections and beliefs of what reality was, or what the truth really was. Evil, inhumanity and violence—could these be examples of what we see in life due to the absence of hope, compassion and acceptance?

One of the conscious decisions that each of us in health care has to be honest with ourselves about is answering the question: To what degree am I my brother's keeper—unconditionally, equivocally or not at all? Taking care of criminals—bad, mean, cruel people—oddly made me return back to my early feelings of knowing that I could not have imagined why some people did what they did to others, so if I had no idea why or how someone chose to do what they did, how then could I judge them?

Awakenings and Lessons Learned

I learned a great deal about my communication patterns, goals, motivations, beliefs, and behaviors. Was this going to help me in my day to day struggles at work? I was silently always wondering this, since going back to school did provide a great distraction from my work life.

Back and forth I went, having experiences that felt ideal in respect to the patients, and then having a series of shifts that resulted in me walking out of the door, thinking "SOS" (Same Old Shit). Why?

I had more lessons to learn.

I realized one very specific type of patient who made me angry were men that spoke to me in a condescending, contemptuous or threatening manner. This felt sexist and demeaning, and though it was often cultural, I at first assumed I didn't like being spoken to in this manner because I had never been treated this way growing up.

I couldn't always walk away from patients or their family members who were vulgar or appeared to want to make me

angry by speaking in a manner that ignited this response in me.
I understood they were in the vulnerable position of being a
patient, of needing my/our help and care, and I usually ignored
a first-time rudely made demand but then I became quite comfortable in saying directly, "Please do not speak to me as you just
did. It is inappropriate. I am here to help you, and I am only
going to tell you this once."

If the behavior continued, it was easy to have a visitor or
family member removed by the full-time security guard or
sheriffs available in every place I have ever worked. If it was the
patient continuing to exert his need for control over me when
he felt powerless because of being a patient, sometimes the only
win was in his wife or daughter witnessing a woman who said,
"No, stop what you are doing," and not getting hurt. I am often
surprised at how one of the tasks of being a nurse is to teach
patients or their family members how to be a patient, or to offer
another communication option and another way of *being*.

The realization that instead of feeling undervalued and not
respected, I realized that I had an unusual opportunity to be a
role model to not this man, BUT to his wife and daughter. I found
that at just this most irritating and demoralizing moment, I did
have the choice not to be a part of some man's power struggle
with a nurse. Did it matter that he probably left the same miserable
person that he was when he came in? No. More importantly, I
had shown his wife and daughter that their worth was not tied to
this man's behavior toward them. Increasingly, these unpleasant
situations were now never reasons for thinking about viewing
nursing as subservient. *I had become the strong nurse I had
fantasized about being when I was young.*

I learned that the pity I felt for some patients had slowly
changed into recognizing that their pain, their suffering was not
a result of being more unfortunate, unlucky or was undeserved.

When I believed that the life some people had been given was *not good enough*, or that it could be better by my standards, I realized that I was still judging their lives.

I thought of people who had experienced severe traumatic accidents, acquired diseases, had less-than-perfect babies, or experienced the death of young children as having *bad lives* until I realized that longevity was not a value of everyone. More was not always better, and a different love was not better than the love you had.

I realized that my learning, as it is with many people, had been focused on completing activities toward what Doctors Ron and Mary Hulnick termed the "goal line" of life (the best schools, the perfect job, making money, acquiring a big home, etc.). However, now I was interested in finding meaning. The "soul line" is concerned with understanding why you are here, not what you have acquired. This belief led me to ask more questions.

- Why had I finally experienced a work environment so difficult, so unsatisfying?
- Why had I stayed for so long?
- What lesson was I there to still learn?

I went through many of my ego-driven beliefs and needs in addition to my judgments of which I was aware and found plenty of "interesting" beliefs I held about myself, my expectations of what I wanted from life and from my profession, and issues related to powerlessness and authority.

The one *type of patient that I had never liked* and had politely fought against was similar to the way I felt about the organization that I now worked for. I felt forced to accept that I was powerless within the organization and powerless when I had to be polite to the occasional male patients that were arrogant, displayed dominant, often not very bright, behaviors, but I had to be respectful to them because I was their nurse. This position of knowing what role, what behaviors I was expected to project as an RN felt similar to the position I felt as an employee within my organization.

Painfully, I had lost respect for the nursing leadership and the realization that I/we were the only ones that this mattered to did not have less merit because we had successfully been ignored.

The nursing care we delivered was often not innovative. It was about actualizing a business or management de jour strategy that reflected a theoretical model by persons that were not going to be present to see if this is what patients wanted, or whose patient experience or outcomes were improved.

> The phrase "nurses eat their young" *used* to mean that older nurses were tough on new nurses. The meaning has expanded.

To my surprise, the distance between nursing leadership and those nurses providing care had not become "more or less" over the years; it remained consistently the same. I realized that the lack of respect I held had been the impedes for my staying, not leaving this workplace. "How you define a problem, is the problem" was a basic belief in my masters program. I now chose to believe that if there had been no issues that needed the attention of the nursing staff, I probably would not have stayed.

This understanding led me to believe that what we needed within my organization, and I now believe is true for other nurses in other organizations, was to continue to seek out the attention and support of our own nursing experts.

The phrase "nurses eat their young" *used* to mean that older nurses were tough on new nurses. This concept still exists but it now pertains to those nurses in leadership that "devour" the nurses that they were intended to advocate for and to lead.

Fighting that had occurred mostly inside myself had not brought about any significant changes at work. Carrying around the heavy armor of being vigilant for battle, looking for further evidence that something might have changed, but never had, for more than twelve years now, had lost meaning to me. Whatever I had hoped to achieve hadn't occurred. This awareness did not bring complete acceptance, but it was a revelation in which I was able to apply to my present work environment. I realized that there was no single "Truth" and "Truth" didn't matter.

... the complex cognitive structure of emotions
has a narrative form—that is that the stories
we tell ourselves are about who we are and
what shapes our emotional and ethical reality is ...
which is the great psychological function of literature.
What emerges is an intelligent manifesto for including
the storytelling arts in moral philosophy.

—MARTHA NUSSBAUM,
PHILOSOPHER, AUTHOR

CHAPTER 20

Defining Our Nobility

Environment plays a big role in influencing
the care provided, but what I learned in my year
that extended to twelve years, was that every day
it was the staff—nurses at all levels, that could
and did overcome ineffective leadership.
Organizational charts did not encourage
communication or practice changes to
bring an institution's "goal statements"
in alignment to the care that patients
actually received.

*"If the only prayer you ever say
in your whole life is 'thank you,'
that would suffice."*
—MEISTER ECKRHART,
Dominican theologian

If nobility is the state of being in one's character, mind,
birthright, rank, associated with dignity, goodness, and
courage, there remained for me the unsettling thought
that there was more to nobility than what nurses provided.

hroughout *The Joy of Nursing* I shared the experiences and reflections that have shaped my life as the nurse, and as the woman that I am today. Over the years, I learned not only how to give care but how diverse the patient experience is. Many in our profession, and those observing us, believe that the nobility of nursing is about the sacrifice, the caring and the sharing of our talents with others. A profession as a whole deserving of the accolade of being described as a "noble" profession is humbling.

Individual nurses have initiated and persevered in bringing about many changes that have contributed to a much more holistic approach to patient wellness. As a professional body, nurses have advanced how care is delivered, supporting individual patients need to find "not just a diagnosis but to find meaning" as they traverse the terrain of illness, healing and health. Knowing that there have been highly significant advances in health care because of nursing still did not quite bring me the closure I was looking for as a bedside nurse.

Being a nurse allowed me the opportunity to witness patients' vulnerability, their struggle to find strength to endure, fight, understand and then accept what was occurring within their own unique worlds. I realized that somehow I had missed that the focus of why I had remained in nursing for so many years, and had been *happy*, even when I had not been, was because it wasn't about what I did for patients, rather it was about what every patient I had cared for brought to our time together.

Nurses bring care; patients bring the nobility.

As nurses we listen to what patients are saying and what they are not saying, as they find their own inner resources to develop answers and meaning to their lives. This is also valuable to us as their care givers. Listening allows for what Mark Nepo refers to as "the silent moments that keep speaking to you" to be heard. In doing so we become open to being fully present with each patient.

Nurses are gifted the opportunity to experience life filled with meaning and purpose because of their role of being a nurse.

Nobility did not come from those of us who chose to provide care to you, and it did not come from our professional designation of being licensed as nurses. The term nobility in conjunction with nursing has always come from the patient. Nurses choose to support and advocate for those persons needing our education, experience, and energy. We believe that our relationship with the patient is based on what we all need from others, and that we will provide compassion when we are at our most vulnerable.

From patients, I found courage, dignity, patience, equanimity and even humor when I needed it, when I felt vulnerable and fearful to life events that occurred to me. At those times in my life, I thought back to patients I had provided care to, and these experiences gifted to me a greater understanding of what *strength, courage* and *dignity* really were.

*No matter how sweet and innocent
your leading characters,
make awful things happen
to them in order that the reader
may see what they are made of.*

—author KURT VONNEGUT's advice to writers

CHAPTER 21

Reclaiming
Our Nobility

The beauty and sacredness of entering
into intimate relationships with strangers
whose names you may never know
is what binds you, the patient, to us,
your nurses.

*Not all complaints are bad,
conflict is normal due to employees
having different strategies based
on their different realities ...*
—JUDITH BRILES, PhD, author, *Stabotage!*

he following excerpt is from the
documentary I wrote and produced,
Exposure: Reclaiming The Nobility of Nursing

"The ritualistic behaviors of preparing to care for patients
are as old as Florence Nightingale's time. As I wash my hands
I find myself thinking that caring for each other represents

the best of our humanness. I began my nursing career 50 years ago, and I have been profoundly moved by the nobility of the nurse-patient relationship of which I have been privileged to be a part, evolving as a nurse, as a person.

Few of us experience life without pain, fear, or loneliness. Few of us are given lives that do not at some time require the care of others. Not knowing what is going to happen when we lose personal control to changes in health, family, finances, or accidents creates vulnerability and fear in us all. These are life's unfolding mysteries, which we all share. Nurses touch these times in people's lives. The beauty and sacredness of entering into intimate relationships with strangers whose names you may never know is what binds you, the patient, to us, your nurses.

My personal search for insight about what it means to be a nurse led me to the startling conclusion that the nobility that has endured for centuries in nursing is currently under the threat of being lost. Lost due to competing and divergent values, goals, and end points from those nurses you have entrusted to provide for you. The essence of our most sacred and trusted promise is one of compassion. Compassion is the response to suffering that patients have always wanted, first and last. I have felt the threat of not always being able to give you the care that I wanted to.

My personal desire to reclaim what I believed was noble about the profession of nursing began with my decision not to pursue a doctorate in nursing. This was my path until I realized that another report on the state of nursing in the twenty-first century was not needed, not from me. I have the utmost admiration and appreciation for the role of advanced-practice nurses and PhD-prepared

nurses who are creating and developing innovative perspectives and strategies to bringing both the complex and
the beautifully needed and wanted value of *caring* to the
fore-front of healing.

Bringing nursing leaders, hands-on nurses, and
academic leaders of our profession closer together—
recognizing that each of these core groups are experts
in their own chosen areas of what it means to be a
nurse—is needed now more than ever!

With a personal career path that has zig-zagged over
the years, I would offer that being in a profession where
there are so many widely variant opportunities, that to
not zig-zag would result in not having taken many of the
opportunities that are available to nurses to grow in
tandem with their own changing wants and needs.

The Reclamation of Joy

But there is work that needs to be done, starting now.

I propose that we start with one very "old" solution that my
fifty years of reflection and in-the-trenches experience brings forth.
I personally believe that this action would positively impact many
of our other professional concerns.

From the beginning of my graduate nursing career in 1971,
I believe that the specific lack of action on what entry into practice
should be represents what has influenced the question as to
whether being a nurse is viewed as a profession or as a career.
Entry into practice has been redefined into a broader meaning
that places the educational preparedness of all levels of nurses
to be the cornerstone of achieving the respect of the physician
staff that we work alongside. To be peers we must be educationally
equivalent. I believe that articulating our separate contributions

at the PhD level is the most important action that will ultimately define that nursing is an unrefuted profession

Nurses realized they possessed a unique and increasingly complex body of knowledge that had become academically, not just clinically, aligned in the 1960s. They also recognized that to be heard, to be invited to upper-level management tables where the power to put into place their ideas was held, they had to become better educated.

As the need for more nurses occurred, this coincided with employing organizations desire to look for ways to decrease overall rising costs of delivering care. Do more with less was the axiom they applied to nursing. The unforeseen but now clearly recognized effect when the need for more nurses was experienced was to churn out more nurses and to educate them with less time and expertise invested in their education.

The paths to becoming an RN have become so diverse that the public and payers for health care services are confused—they don't know what to expect.

Research has been conducted to provide information regarding the substitution of registered nurses with less-educated staff members, and it is occurring insidiously in many sites. Health care is being leveraged by hiring freezes bolstered by the falsehood, "You did okay being one nurse down from your previous level of staffing, we will *allow* you to rehire into your vacant position in three months ... in six months ...".

Angry nurses do not choose to be angry.

Registered nurses understand that the decision to utilize less-educated nurses as a means to keeping personnel costs down will always look attractive and be supported by management. Even if *they resist* and even if *they groan,* "get them to come in and work" is the strategy that has worked for a long time.

"Voting with your feet," choosing to stay or leave a work environment based on your values aligning with your employer, remains the strongest action nurses can take. Nursing represents the largest workforce in the delivery of health care. The need to ensure that there is choice in care environments such that *not* the most financially motivated systems price out more patient-centered environments will only occur if those sites that are struggling to fight their systems that are looking for the least prepared, least expensive workforce, is seen as successful by those places still valuing an educated, well-paid workforce.

Nurses in these sites practice what is often referred to as "work-arounds." To some degree someone must be responsible to recognize and fill the gaps that are a byproduct of our complex healthcare system. Patients fall into the fragmented cracks of our highly complex systems within systems of health care. Dr. Jean Watson challenges nursing to reflect on what "carative" behaviors are unique to nursing and not to abdicate from them. Her science of caring is an excellent example of evidence-based positive outcomes to patient care, but the desire and need to incorporate these carative activities by nurses can be difficult to achieve.

Novelist Toni Morrison reflected that history is important:
> The past is rife with values worthy of reverence and transmission … [but] the past is already in debt to the mismanaged present. And, besides, contrary to what you may have heard or learned, the past is not done and it is not over, it's still in process, which is another way of saying that when it's critiqued, analyzed, it yields new information about itself. The past is already changing as it is being reexamined, as it is being listened to for deeper resonances.

With all that we know about the historical *whys* of this profession's subservience, in conjunction with the strong, truly valuable contributions to improving the health of people who needed more than a *cure* (especially when a cure is not on the table), we may be rated high on respectability surveys comparing occupations, but registered nurses are being replaced with other nurse look-alikes and in some cases, wannabes.

- We need solutions to be offered not because they are error free when they are first proposed but because they encourage others to get out of their professional silos.

- We need to consider a solution that may sound outrageous or impossible but, with collaborative work, might be just what the profession needs.

We know that we've made innovative inroads in creating exciting, autonomous, highly valued roles for nurses, but these roles are not sufficient enough to replace the number of exiting nurses.

Disgruntled nurses must be heard; dialogues of discontent encouraged. There needs to be dialogue among the pillars of academia, leadership and the hands-on nurses. I remember thinking that maybe there were some "negative nurses out there with bad attitudes," until I looked like one of these nurses, years into my career!

I know many, many nurses. Some have been close friends for decades, some are recent friends while others are acquaintances or I *know* them through their blogs or publications. Each of these nurses has something different to say about our field, depending upon his or her experience. We are all guardians of our patients' nobility; it is up to us.

We chose this profession, not because of its problems. How we resolve the problems will define us.

- We need the diversity and the input of people in nursing who *look like* all of us. Each community, culture, country has a "face" there is comfort in receiving care by someone that feels like where we have come from.

- The profession needs the most innovative problem solvers, people committed to mending the suffering of humanity.

> "Is nursing something one is called to do?" I am often asked. My answer has always been "If you're lucky."

For those looking for one of the most purposeful ways to live a life, never wondering what meaning your life has, that is exactly what being a nurse offers.

To be a nurse answers the most fundamental question that unites us all:

Why am I here?

What is my unique destiny to fulfill?

Have we listened, and do we know how patients desire to feel cared for, or how they define health and wholeness?

Do we assume we know that longevity is always best, or that we know patients' deepest fears, or how, if their ends are imminent, they want to live, if we don't have time to ask them?

More than ever, to heal, one has to feel cared for, but with all of the technology and medical options so abundant, we need people who have chosen alternative ways to live, inviting new definitions of health to encourage greater patient participation.

"I'll bet you've seen it all," I hear all of the time, but I still haven't. It took decades of being a nurse to realize I had seen many dramatic, one-of-a-kind experiences and been witness to extraordinary events in people's lives, and for this, my *work* was not work ... it was *Joy*.

Thirty years into my career, while filming my documentary *Exposure: Reclaiming the Nobility of Nursing*, I thought I knew where I was going when I started, but I ended up in a completely unexpected place. *Exposure* was about 20 nurses spanning 30 years: my colleagues and me and the many exposures and situations we experienced. I realized that the title I had selected for this documentary was actually a metaphor for my exposure, not exposing nursing to others, but to myself. It was my *own exposure* to the toughness and the tenderness of nursing, not of the *doing*, but of the *being* with patients,

I realized that I share a kinship with nurses wherever I've traveled around the world. "We get a lot of thanks from our patients, but we also get a whole lot back from them," Pam long ago shared in the filming of *Exposure*.

"Is nursing something one is called to do?" I am often asked. My answer has always been, "If you're lucky." I believe that if you are a patient, you will most likely want what I want.

- *I want to know* I will be treated kindly, competently, with respect for my body, my thoughts, and my feelings, especially when I am unable to take care of myself.

- *I want to trust* you to listen to me and be available to be patient or firm with me.

- *I want to believe* you will not judge me when I am not at my best, and you will be hopeful for me and truthful to me as I experience the destiny before me.

- *I am hopeful* that my nurse will invite me to express myself and possibly put my needs and wants before those to whom I have entrusted my life, even if we may not be in agreement as to what is *best* for me.

We are all in the process of healing. This path is a lifelong inner journey. Being open to the suffering of others opens us to our own suffering. Compassion is not something I can give to someone; rather it is the sharing of who we each authentically are. Our shared humanity is not based on who *gives* and who *receives* care.

My patients and I have a relationship in which healing the woundedness of bodies and hearts does not occur because of hospitals, religions, doctors, nurses, or what any of us do. Healing is not just the absence of disease or fixing someone wherever or whenever we meet to heal. The language of healing is love. We have within us the resources to transform humanity by being the divineness that we all are right now.

Joy had come from pain. Joy had come from reflecting on choosing to become who I needed to be. I had a vision of what being a nurse was and this guided me to bring this presence to the to the patients I provided care.

The great big world
that might have grown small to you,
though it is right where you left it …
asks, you have the keys—
don't you want to use them?

—AUTHOR UNKNOWN

CHAPTER 22

AfterWord

A young patient was heard saying this to a
nurse somewhere, was how I was told this story:
"When I grow up, I want to be just like you."
"A nurse?"
"No, I want to be an angel."

*"Mom, as a beginning second-year
medical student, I feel like the nurses are the
ones who know everything about the patients.
I had no idea that they knew so much".*
—AINSLEY ADAMS

*ow did this daughter of ours become so
smart?* I smiled inwardly to myself and
fist-pumped a righteous, "Yes!"
There were so many great experiences that I have had as a
nurse. I have continued to work in Ambulatory Care as there is
still much work that needs the confidence and conviction that I
look for in proactive, non-overly compromising nursing leadership, but especially with every new graduate nurse that I meet.

We need your ideals, your vision, your lack of experience, your beliefs that are based on no experience but lots of hope.

Hands-on patient care should be THE "product line!" Putting meaning into the phrase that "patients are the center of why we are here," must be believed by those that have direct patient contact.

The increasing opportunities for nurses along with the aging of a large percentage of nurses currently in practice has created a shortage of nurses in some geographical and patient care areas. This shortage of nurses, is arguable to some degree. But, there is agreement that attracting new, younger nurses is necessary and needed.

In the next five years many nurses of my generation will retire. It is my hope that passing information on from *those of us close to exiting the profession* will enrich your practice. *The Joy of Nursing, Reclaiming Our Nobility* was written to provide a viewpoint—a candid portrayal of the profession.

- *Challenge yourself. Come be a nurse with us*
- *There are problems and they need the input that possibly only you can provide!*

I often say this to groups that I am addressing.

I have confidence that you will be there to provide excellent care to us. The increasing number of older persons coupled with the ever increasing new technological options you will be expected to learn are challenges that you do have the resiliency, tenacity and creativity to translate into excellent patient care. I know this because you follow the generations of nurses that have come before you and have been there for their patients.

February 2015

I was looking for a data reference while working on this manuscript and I found the following email, dated six years earlier from my nurse friend Anne.

> *Julie … Remember that little girl that looked like your Ainsley that we were both so upset about years ago? I'm surprised that we never talked about her and it made me wonder, did I forget to tell you that one of the social workers came in six months later and told me that she had been adopted by a really loving and remarkable couple.*

I couldn't believe what I was reading!

I had never seen this email. Yet here it was, here it had been for six years.

This little girl had haunted me for years.

Tears, relief and peace … for *The Joy of Nursing*.

Go home to yourself.

—MITCH ROSACKER

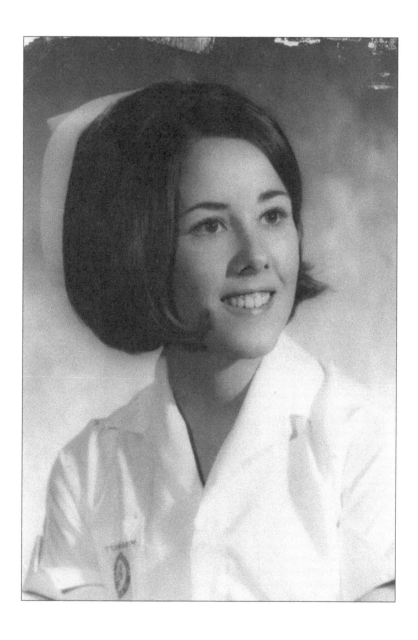

About the Author

JULIANA ADAMS, BSN, MSN, MA is part of a unique number of nurses who have dedicated more than a half century to the care of patients ... and to the advancement of the nursing profession. She remains actively engaged in how nursing care is delivered.

She is an author, speaker and film maker.

Juliana divides her time between Englewood, Colorado and Steamboat Springs, Colorado. She and her husband, along with pets left by their two children who are pursuing their own admirable dreams, have chosen to work in their respective fields, for many years to come.

JulianaAdamsInc@gmail.com

JulianaAdamsInc.com

 www.facebook.com/JulianaAdamsAuthor1

 www.linkedin.com/in/julianaadams

Working with
Juliana Adams

COMPLAINING, BLAMING, LOOKING THE OTHER WAY takes energy. Energy that is lost.

Juliana Adams has been there.

Getting good at being stuck can occur at staff and leadership levels in any organization.

When there is discord, apathy or anger in a work environment, it can be easy for the emotional responses that build up regarding long term conflict, to be judged as bad. These feelings can masquerade as facts.

As nurses, we can slip into victimhood, just as leaders can believe they are solving problems. Recognizing that our own personal judgment of what is "right" is often what separates us.

Dialogues of discontent need not perpetrate negativism. They can powerfully open doors and promote moving from rhetoric to meaningful results.

In her presentations, Juliana invites nurses to understand, in a new uplifting manner, the concepts of:

PRIDE	COMPETING MISSION
VALUE	MAKING A DIFFERENCE
TRUTH	FINDING MEANING
RESPECT	CELEBRATING THE JOY OF NURSING

She invites nurses at all levels to rethink their own personal frustrations, anger or disillusionment; replacing self-limiting beliefs with a personal invitation to discover the joy of what being a nurse means to you. Juliana will excite her audiences to live their inspired self.

As a guest speaker or panelist, she creates an environment of acceptance for what may begin with differing perspectives, but will result in each participant valuing the care that they uniquely provide. Juliana Adams provides to you and your organization:

- Shifting negativity and burnout to novel approaches for feeling valued and connected to the organization. *The Joy of Nursing.*

- How to be more than the conductor on the train ... Empowerment is personal.

- Being comfortable with being uncomfortable ... Our own and our patients' sources of angst.

- Looking beyond the diagnosis ... the face behind the case and your nurse is more than "just a nurse."

- Competing missions may feel like they exist in nursing today ... How to find peace with conflicting values and directives.

- Where does the nobility in nursing come from?

Remember the joy of saying:

"I am your nurse and I am here to make things better."

Contact Juliana at | 720-488-6914 | JulianaAdamsInc@gmail.com

Acknowledgments

*S*torytellers have given me gifts of themselves that took me places, and brought forward meanings that I never would have come to on my own. These people lit up my imagination and became life threads of inspiration.

My *Dream Team* from USM: Delores, Shirley and Carol: we made a great team who did accomplish our shared mission of assisting each other to produce original courageous expressions of who we were on the inside, but what had not yet made it to the *outside*. My documentary: *Exposure, Reclaiming the Nobility of Nursing* came from our time together, and led me to *The Joy of Nursing, Reclaiming Our Nobility*.

The women in the National League of American Pen Women-Denver were the first people to read my book draft. Their encouragement and expertise as authors taught me that all writers must persevere with endless rewrites, till you simply *get it right*. Ruthy Denker, who I first met when I was captivated by her writing, and then by her. She took my story and me under her wing and taught me the power of *showing, not telling*. Ruthy, Kelly Ann, Diane, Donna, Kay and Kathleen—my critique group. Thank you for your patience and encouragement.

To Dr. Jody who prepared me for Dr. Judith Briles, whose expertise and motivational persona is better and more real than her world-wide reputation. Her wit and her intensity have kept her on the top of the publishing world for two decades and the phrase, "How do you think people made it to the top of the mountain, they weren't just dropped off there," comes to mind every time she pushed for me.

To my incredible family—each of whom offered me special encouragement. To Braden for always asking, "How's the book going, Mom" month after month. To Ainsley who said, "I'm so impressed. You wrote that chapter in the dark, in the back seat of the car, with a flashlight" as we drove to the Great Smoky Mountains prior to Braden's deployment to Afghanistan. And to my darling husband Bruce who I kiddingly say is "the love and money guy." You remained by my side on so many late, late nights working on endless re-edits of my documentary and my book. I can never say I love you enough, or thank you enough, honey! And when you say, "I'd do it all over again," I melt.

My brother Perry Hackett and friend Debby Bess, you are my "family," and treasures to me. You both remember stories about when I first said, "I want to be a nurse." Thank you.

To Mitch Rosacker who taught me to listen to myself and *To Go There and Roam* when I felt desperate to believe in myself but needed to be shown the way when it felt too risky to do this alone.

Erica, thank you for dropping your stuff to help me with fonts, color and confidence. Your company, ThistleSociety.com will produce beautifully feminine and demure clothing!

To Pam, "Star Maker and Star," and all of my fellow nurses at the DG ER "back then" and who are, amazingly still in my life. It was *Camelot Nursing* being with you: the two Donnas, Meredith, Lulu, Toni, Vickie A., Vickie O., Georgia, Kathy, Cathy, Becky, Debby K., Debbie J., Carolee, Judy, Liz, Anne and Marion.

To my friend Melody who was given a life full of events as a mother, wife, woman and patient, that would have taken most people past their breaking point years ago. She falls to her knees and asks God to be with her to show her how strong and loving she needs to be for the many people whose lives depend on her. In total admiration, thank you for teaching me that love, just as it is, is enough.

Norma, Heide, Connie and Pattie E you are the best friends! Growing old with you has got to be as neat as staying young together has been!

A big thank you to Rebecca Finkel for all of her flexibility and patience, over and over again when it must have seemed like my book would never get finished.

To the nurses I currently work with who provide care that often goes far beyond the extra mile to put patients' needs first. In the end, working with you was a Nursing Camelot time in my life. You make a difference in patients lives every shift, by making endless *work-arounds* to keep patients safer and feeling cared for. Nurses like these nurses are the safety net within healthcare delivery systems throughout America.

Nurses go to work every day to make a difference in patients' lives, making endless work-arounds to keep patients safer and feeling cared for. To all patients that may have felt invisible, fearful or alone in their journey to find meaning when they have needed healing. As nurses we know that you need our hope, compassion and competency. We seek to ensure that your voice is heard. I humbly speak for the many, many nurses I have worked with for more than fifty years, by expressing to you that we consider our relationship with you sacred.